the Patient's and the Doctor's Dilemma
THE ROSEBUD STORY

By

DR ROXANA CHAPMAN

Barham Press

2007

Dedication

To my parents who gave me the gift of life and nurtured me, and to my loving family (my husband and my two sons).

Acknowledgements

I owe an immense debt of gratitude to my patients who became not only my teachers but also my friends, and who permitted, and encouraged me to write this book. They shared with me their inmost thoughts, with the realization that, although they themselves would not benefit from it, yet with the belief that their stories might be of help to others who might find themselves in a similar predicament.

I am grateful to my two dear sons, David and Harold, who, far from begrudging the many extra hours that I devoted to my patients rather than to them, actually encouraged me to publish this precious collection of medical case histories collected over the course of some thirty-seven years. In addition to this, however,they both read through the entire manuscript and made useful comments or gave alternative suggestions so that it would be more comprehensible for the non-medical readers for whom it was mainly written.

I thank my darling husband, Dr Kenneth, for his psychological, scientific and spiritual help throughout our medical careers, and for his practical help and advice during the writing of this book.

Finally, I am particularly grateful to our dear friend and colleague, Professor Marius Plouzhnikov, who not only supplied me with much statistical data from Russia, but who allowed me to include one of the true stories that he has written.

Introduction

He who looks to the past is in danger of losing an eye.
He who ignores the past is in danger of losing both eyes.
Russian Proverb

S ecret and silent voices whisper through the pages of this book. They have told their simple, yet often harrowing stories to arouse compassion, but also to stimulate and to educate.

These women, of different races, nationalities, social classes and religions all have one thing in common: they have all been faced with the perplexing choice of whether or not to undergo termination of pregnancy. They come from women who have undergone life-changing experiences and are brave enough to share them with others. Such stories as are recounted in this book may be challenging, frustrating, sometimes exciting or exhilarating, but always illuminating.

I myself, am a female gynaecologist, who has practised my chosen specialty in several different countries around the world, and for the last fifteen years in London. I have been greatly privileged that so many of my patients have confided their most intimate thoughts to me, and that several have begged me to publish their histories in the hope that other women may learn from their ordeals and have the courage to apply what they have learnt.

Pro-life and pro-choice antagonists have argued, often violently, about the ethical and practical issues of abortion for at least 2,500 years, often without having any first hand experience of the conflicting motives which may arise for those unfortunately faced by stark choices. Hundreds of books have been written by the supporters of a particular point of view. It is hoped that both camps may learn from those courageous women who have bared their souls and have thus enabled this book to be written.

Most people agree that we learn by experience but fewer hold to the belief that the lessons of history can help us to avoid making the same mistakes in the future. They may pay lip service to such a belief but their subsequent actions belie their protestations.

The Consulting Room has always been a place of fascination and mystery for people, resembling, as it does, the Confessional of the Priest, and for similar reasons. It has been my great privilege, not only to listen to the stories recorded in the following pages, but also to have been given permission and, indeed, encouraged by some of the participants to make known to a wider public their inmost feelings, struggles and temptations. Such records are priceless, and I offer them to the reader to study each history and to draw his or her own conclusions.

This book is not a novel. It is a collection of case histories that are recorded so that others might learn from them. I encountered many rocks and rapids during my own voyage of discovery so I think it would be helpful if I recount a little of my own struggles at the beginning of the book.

Foreword

The author's presentation is indeed a moving account of her experience in the complexities in the field of abortion. Her prime concern in preserving life is well illustrated in the "Abortionist's Story".

As an ex-paediatric colleague of Dr Chapman I recall her total dedication in the field of Obstetrics and her concern in the follow up of newborn babies.

The evolution in the field of diagnostic tests in utero and the ability in treating certain congenital defects is testimony to her altruistic attitude in preserving life throughout her full medical career.

Dr Beryl Banner, former colleague and paediatrician

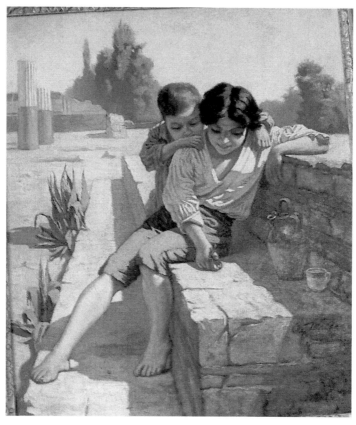

Painted by Alexander Maclean in 1893.

For he comes, the human child,
    To the waters and the wild
With a faery, hand in hand,
    For the world's more full of weeping
than he can understand.

William Butler Yeats

Table of Contents

Table of Contents continued

Headings   Pages

Abortion;

the Patient's and the Doctor's dilemma

The Rosebud Story

Derivation of the Title

Iloved every aspect of Medical School, even if I found some things unpleasant, such as working in the Dissecting Room on dead bodies, because I realised that it was necessary in order that I might fully understand the anatomy of the human body and so become a good clinician. However the day came when we were studying the functions of the body in Physiology that we were told that we would shortly be carrying out experiments on living animals, such as frogs, mice and rats. This I found very difficult to accept because I loved animals and had, during my childhood years, gathered a large quantity of animals around me, indeed a veritable zoo! I was as a child fascinating to study animal behaviour, for one observed their fear, as well as their affection and loyalty. I could even, I thought, understand a little of their language. Not, of course, like Dr Dolittle, but anyone who has brought up a baby animal from birth develops a bond with it, analogous to that of a mother who understands her baby and its needs before it can talk.

I have many stories that I could tell about the care of animals for their young offspring. The most amazing was that of 'my' horse who disappeared from her paddock when heavily pregnant. She foaled in the wild and must have protected her young foal from wolves for about a week before she was found. During that time she could barely have eaten or drunk anything, because she was in the last stages of dehydration and hunger when she was found and taken home. There she collapsed and looking at her young foal, her eyes filled with tears, and she expired. I could only have been about three at the time, but the scene will be forever in my memory.

Thus, being very sensitive to the feelings and pain of animals and knowing that I had to participate in animal research, I took with me a book of poetry and a pair of scissors, sat myself down in my parents' rose garden in Iran and started to cut off the buds on all the rose bushes. In that way, perhaps, I thought I might be brave enough to participate in the forthcoming physiological experiments:

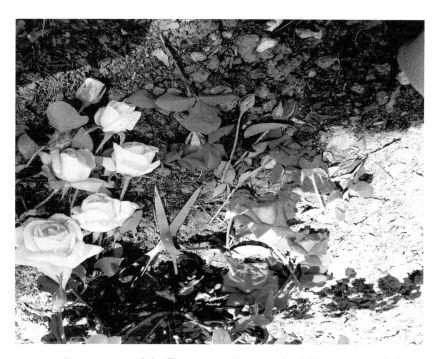

Sweet rose, fair flower, untimely pluck'd, soon vaded,
Pluck'd in the bud, and vaded in the spring!
Bright orient pearl alack! Too timely shaded;
Fair creature, kill'd too soon by death's sharp sting!
W. Shakespeare

The Hippocratic Oath

I come from a medical family and I remember as a small child rescuing flies and other insects from a pond in the garden and trying to resuscitate them, since I believed that that was the main purpose of being a doctor. It never even occurred to me that payment would be expected, but of course, at that stage of my existence, food, clothing and all other requirements necessary for living were supplied free of charge and apparently spontaneously.

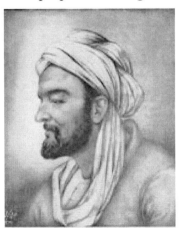

Avicenna, Doctor of doctors

My parents, noting my growing interest in things medical, showed me when I was considerably older, that great encyclopaedic book of Avicenna, "The Qunun". Written in the 11th century it was later translated into Latin and soon occupied a place of pre-eminence in Western medical literature, displacing such famous works as those of Galen. Avicenna thus became my hero and I longed to enter medical school and follow in his footsteps.

At medical school I became familiar with another medical giant of antiquity, Hippocrates. This acquaintanceship became

3

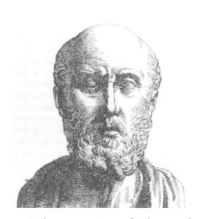

Hippocrates, father of medicine

more meaningful when, as graduands, we subscribed to a modified version of the Hippocratic Oath in which we promised to treat our patients to the best of our ability, to abstain from doing them mischief, not to carry out abortions on any women, and not to divulge anything that we might hear or see during such attendance.

It is one of the oldest binding documents in history, and has remained as the guideline of medical ethics for doctors for the past 2,400 years. Hippocrates realized that a patient's willingness to trust his or her physician was essential for the practice of medicine. Without such trust medicine could neither flourish nor progress, and, from the patient's perspective, it represented the guarantee of his or her freedom and liberty.

This concept of medicine has remained with me throughout my medical career. For this reason I was reluctant to write this book, in spite of the fact that some of my patients had asked me to tell their stories so that others could avoid making the same mistakes. However, the abortion controversy is as hotly debated as it ever was, and I have therefore written down a few of the many case histories that I have collected over the course of many years, with names and sometimes locations altered to protect patients' identities, in the hope that it will contribute to the debate.

Early Experiences — Pro-choice

lthough I was born in Persia to parents who loved each other dearly I fairly soon was able to appreciate that the country in which I lived was a male dominated one. The women folk's lives very much depended upon the whims and preferences of their male partners. Servants too were treated with little regard, more especially if they happened to be of the female gender. Thus, at quite an early age I began to call for the rights of women to be respected, and it motivated me to enter the army as an officer, to train as an army doctor, and to fight for, and to achieve, equality in rank and position with the men.

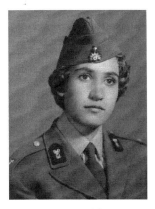

Dr Roxana Chapman
as army officer

While I was a medical student, I remember being put in charge of a young girl of 16 who was having a baby. She refused a vaginal examination and told me that she was a virgin and wanted to keep it that way. I said, "But you're pregnant!" She replied "The man who made me pregnant told me that he would not alter my virginity." She was then in the second stage of labour, was screaming with pain, and trying to sit on the baby's head to prevent it from being born. I learnt subsequently that she was a simple, country girl who had been employed as a servant by a wealthy couple. They had a grown up, sexually promiscuous son whom they hoped to protect from visiting prostitutes by taking into service a poor, ignorant girl who would, they hoped, act as an unwitting concubine. I was incensed.

I suppose that, in spite of my desire for the rights of women to be respected, I remained rather innocent and oblivious of the deviousness of human nature for several years, until well after I had become a doctor. We had, of course, studied embryology at medical school, but pictures in a textbook meant little when compared with the real life drama of working in a dissecting room in the anatomy department, and I really had little idea of the incidence of criminal abortion, nor of the appearance of an early foetus.

After completing my studies I came to work in London and I remember being on call one night during my first houseman's appointment and being summoned to see a patient who was brought in bleeding vaginally. I examined her and found that the vagina was badly ulcerated and that there was, what appeared to be, a small hole in the upper vagina through which blood was trickling. I had already taken a history but the woman obviously was not telling me the full story. Taking out my emergency vademecum (medical handbook) I scanned the pages but soon found that I could make nothing of it. I therefore admitted her to the ward and called the registrar. He told me that it was an attempted abortion. He gave her a course of antibiotics, packed the vagina, and told me that she appeared to be about twelve weeks pregnant.

The following day she told me everything. Her husband, who was twice her age, had children from a previous marriage and did not want any more. He insisted that he could not afford more children and took her to a back street abortionist who poured potassium permanganate into her vagina. The burning pain was intense and she left the abortionist in terrible distress. As this did not terminate the pregnancy her husband insisted that she should return to the abortionist. She, however, could not face to see the abortionist again, so decided to attempt herself to end the pregnancy herself with a knitting needle. This she hesitatingly did, but there was a sudden sharp pain, and then she started to bleed heavily. She begged me not to write what she had told me in her notes in case her husband got into trouble.

The patient herself haled from Romania where she had lived a sad, impoverished life. Eventually she was brought to this country with a family to act as their nanny. Here she looked after the children and did all the housework. She loved children. That indeed was why she agreed to become a nanny, with the hope that one day she would marry, as indeed she did, and have children of her own. This was to be her first child. She did not miscarry. Instead, she carried her pregnancy to term and delivered a healthy baby. Her husband gave her no support. Instead, he abandoned her. My heart went out to that woman. She was only twenty-four, the same age as myself.

During the following six months I was on duty in the Casualty Department of a London hospital once a week, and rarely one of those evenings passed without me having to admit a woman who had attempted to do away with her unborn child. Such an introduction to the woes of many workingwomen, together with my compassion, when a child, for the downtrodden women of my own country, made me anxious to fight for the rights of women.

I was also appalled that so many men, as it appeared to me, withdrew from a relationship as soon as the wife or girlfriend became pregnant, and left the poor, unfortunate woman to face the future alone. It appeared that the man was not considered to bear any responsibility for his action. Where was the justice in that? If the woman was denied the right to choose then, it seemed to me, she was denied the right to control her own body. All this misery made me anxious to fight for the rights of women and I even took part in a march to lobby Parliament. I did not believe that a government should be allowed to trample on the individual's personal rights of freedom, since at that time abortion was illegal.

In those days I thought that women only had terminations in cases of rape, incest, chronic and serious health conditions, or if made to have abortions by vicious and uncaring husbands. I thought that the decision was a private matter between the woman and her doctor and that the doctor always knew best. I was strongly against private abortion clinics and believed that they should be performed in public hospitals, free of charge. Besides campaigning for women's rights I also campaigned for financial help to be given by the government to poor women who wished to keep their babies. Basically, I believed in the woman's right to choose, and to have reproductive freedom. Obviously, it will be seen by those who have read what I have written that, at that time, my beliefs were very confused and contradictory. Truly, our lives are shaped by what we see, by what we are told, by our early beliefs, by the society that we grew up in, by the school to which we were sent, and by the books that we read. All play a part in perfecting or spoiling our character.

All that was to change when I was working as a senior house officer during my first gynaecological appointment. A woman who had been admitted for a 'Dilatation and Curettage' (obtaining scrapings from the lining of the womb for diagnostic purposes) continued to bleed. I had not been looking after her but since I was on duty I went to see her. I carried out an internal examination and was shocked, indeed, horrified to feel a tiny baby's hand in the vagina. "You were pregnant!" I screamed. "No, I wasn't." she replied. Her denial, and the duplicity of the doctor who had admitted her for a 'D & C' stunned me. The scales fell from my eyes and I realised, for the first time, that an abortion consisted of the dismembering of a living human being, and was not, as the media was pleased to say, the scraping out of a few cells and some blood.

My eyes having been opened to the realities of abortion, I should like to conclude by portraying some of the delights of child birth and motherhood: As a girl of eighteen entering medical school I was particularly dismayed by the bulging abdomen and slovenly appearance of pregnant women, by the screaming in the delivery ward, and by their subsequently stretched, scarred abdomens. This initially put me off midwifery and everything connected with it. However, some years later when still a student, while looking after a Japanese patient in labour and noticing her anguish with each contraction, I suggested to her that she should accept some pain-relief. Noticing that I was young and inexperienced she replied, "Why do you think some people run twenty-six miles in a marathon? They suffer much pain and exhaustion during the race, but at the end, they get great joy and a feeling of achievement. It's the same with having a baby. I don't want my exhilaration ruined by being made semi-conscious." This put an entirely new picture on the case and I began to see that pregnancy and childbirth, far from being a blot on the human predicament, was perhaps its crowning glory.

Thereafter obstetrics became, for me, a much more attractive profession which culminated in the birth of my first son. It was a really wonderful, indeed, a spiritual experience. Although an obstetric colleague of mine agreed to be available for my delivery, nevertheless, I preferred to have my husband, himself a consultant obstetrician and gynaecologist, to conduct the second stage of labour, and I relied entirely upon him to deliver our child. Nothing in the world can compare with the joy and happiness experienced by a mother when she gives birth to her child, more especially when it is her first, and this happiness is shared by all in any way connected with the birth: the husband, the waiting relatives, and even the midwives and nurses in the labour ward. When I had my children it was not customary for a husband to be anywhere near the labour ward. Thank God nowadays husbands are encouraged to be present, and even to assist in the birthing process, if it only be to give encouragement. It must surely help in the bonding, and this is the more important nowadays when both parents often go out to work and the husband is more frequently left in charge of the developing child.

If the birth of a baby gives so much happiness how can it be that so many women seek termination of their unborn child? One can understand the terror and sense of helplessness of a young, unmarried girl, but less so of a happily married woman. It was a great shock to me when I first beheld doctors carrying out abortions. Many did them unwillingly and I remember when I refused to carry them out that one doctor said to me, "Why do you leave us to do your dirty work?" Why, if they knew that it was 'dirty work', did they themselves agree to perform the terminations? Other doctors, of course, without such scruples, sought employment in private abortion clinics where they could earn much more money than they could in the National Health Service. Those seeking Consultant status in Obstetrics and Gynaecology in the N.H.S. were always asked by the interviewing committee if they would agree to perform abortions (although the Government always denied that this occurred) and if they did not agree they would not be appointed. Thus, in the process of time, all N.H.S. hospitals came to be staffed by obstetricians who were prepared to carry out the Government's remit to terminate pregnancies as requested.

The Doctors' Lounge

It was early morning when I finished my night duty in the newborn intensive care unit, or the Special Care Baby Unit (SCBU) as it was officially called. The sun began to shine on the tall buildings and the high trees that surrounded the hospital. The air was fresh and a soft breeze was blowing. After the tension of the night I felt that a stroll in the nearby park would relax me sufficiently to enable me to concentrate on my duties in the clinic which were due to start in one and a half hours' time. The park was beautiful. The blackbirds were singing in the lilacs, and a slight mist arose from the ground before being dispersed by the rising sun.

The activities that took place in SCBU still filled my mind. The neonatal unit was quite different from almost every other hospital department, caring, as it does, for ill, or newborn, premature babies. For parents it can often be the most stressful and traumatic episode in their lives thus far, and even the doctors and nurses can find it harrowing. Most junior doctors in SCBU are competent, and, although they feel the surge of adrenaline (a hormone produced by the adrenal gland that causes a rise of blood-pressure and equips the animal or human being for fight or flight) as they struggle to deal with some neonatal complication, nevertheless, find the experience both beneficial and rewarding. They see the very beginnings of human life outside the womb, and are enabled to empathise with the anxious parents.

Much sophisticated equipment is needed for the care of these very small babies. All are nursed in incubators. Most are attached to various types of monitor, and some require respiratory support with extra oxygen to maintain a continuous positive airway pressure. These, together with all the other essential equipment required to furnish the department, cost many thousands of pounds.

As I walked further in the park I reached a pond where several waterfowl were swimming. Amongst them was a proud mother duck with her seven tiny offspring. I was still thinking of my time in the premature baby unit and wondered if animals sometimes had premature babies. I thought of all the physiological variables such as heart rate, blood pressure, respiration rate, and oxygen and carbon dioxide levels in the blood. Some needed to be checked or sampled every few seconds so that the clinician, in conjunction with the laboratory responsible for the various blood or serum analyses, could make the correct decision for best treatment.

Time was running out so I retraced my steps to the hospital and entered the doctors' sitting room where I hoped that I should find the registrar or consultant, for I wished to ask a question about an extremely premature baby whom I had been looking after during the preceding night. I had, of course, handed over the care of the premature babies to someone else before I left the department, but as a junior doctor, one was always anxious to learn more.

For those of you who do not know what a doctors' lounge or sitting room is, it is worth pointing out that when the National Health Service was first founded the junior doctors lived as a community and were provided with bedrooms, dining room and sitting room where they slept, ate and relaxed when not working. Consultants, too, were welcomed in the sitting room and dining room and much of the care of patients was discussed and arranged over a cup of tea or during a meal.

Not immediately seeing the person I was looking for I decided to relax, have a cup of coffee and, perhaps find in my paediatric textbook an answer to my query. I was quite anxious about that tiny, twenty-two-week-old who was fighting for his life. Morbidity and mortality are so high in those tiniest of babies that if one makes the slightest mistake the consequences can be devastating, if not fatal. Not only that, but the babies' parents have put their faith and trust in the hospital staff and, if for no other reason, it is our duty to do the best we can.

Eventually the registrar arrived for a pre-clinic coffee, and I approached him with my mug of coffee in my hand. Some other resident doctors were there, either glancing at the morning papers, talking about a play or concert they had attended the night before, or, more usually, discussing patients in their care.

Suddenly my attention was arrested by hearing a locum consultant obstetrician and gynaecologist speaking about a late termination that she had just carried out. The 1967 Abortion Act had fairly recently been implemented so I was curious to hear what she was saying. She had been a Medical Missionary in Africa, but had now returned to this country. She was saying loudly, as though seeking advice or assistance, "I had to abort a 24-week-old twin pregnancy early this morning. The babies were so strong, and were crying so loudly, that I didn't know what to do. Eventually I had to bash their heads to shut them up." Every one looked at her in horror. I really did not know what I was hearing and, for a second, I thought that she had attacked some of the babies in the intensive care unit. What if someone had attacked the 22-week-old baby whom I had been looking after? I was young and tender hearted. What I had just heard made me feel sick, and I was overcome by a cold sweat.

The doctor stopped talking when she realized that what she was saying was upsetting those who were present. Was it a cri de coeur? How could a missionary doctor behave in such a way? Did she believe that now the Abortion Act was law she was bound to obey its every dictate? Or did she think that she was helping the woman who, not wanting any more babies, had demanded the termination? I said to myself, "How can that doctor speak so boldly in front of everyone?" I wanted to rush and rescue those babies; but it was too late. They were dead.

What was the logic in trying to preserve the life of a 22-week-old baby in one part of the hospital when, in another part, two even larger babies were having their lives taken? If I, through negligence, brought about the death of a baby who was in my care, I might well be taken to court and tried for manslaughter. On the other hand, the law permits me at the mother's request, and with the approval of two doctors, to kill even larger babies with impunity. The same law, the same country, the same people; the sense of injustice remains with me to this day.

As an obstetrician I have two patients to consider: the mother and the child that she is carrying, and during my training I learnt, not only the skills required, but developed a love and compassion for the tiny baby for whom I was responsible. The baby also is given rights and the law permits him/her to sue me for negligence up to his/her age of twenty-one years. Babies are now surviving at 21 or 22 weeks and are given the protection of the law. What of those late abortions, often older than 21 weeks? The law is inconsistent, and if young doctors witness the duplicity of their mentors and lose their compassion, humanity will be the poorer.

Power-cut and Blackout in London

Blackout during the Second World War was still fresh in the minds of those who had lived through it when, some twenty-five or so years later, industrial action led to massive strikes which caused power cuts, chaos and major disruption in people's lives. Rail and tube services came to a halt. Trains and stations were plunged into darkness with some passengers actually being trapped under-ground when the power was switched off.

Hospitals did not escape the chaos. Many doctors and nurses either did not manage to get to work or, if they were at work, failed to get home at the end of their shifts. This added considerably to the strain of hard-pressed medical and nursing staff who were present in the hospitals. They were responsible for the lives of their patients who were also put at risk in the minute or minutes that elapsed before hospital generators were able to take over. This was particularly the case in Intensive Care Units where ventilators had to be managed by hand before the hospital generators started up. In some parts of the hospital, indeed, some staff struggled to keep going with the aid of candle or battery power,

Limited supplies from stand-by generators kept premature babies alive, stocks of blood useable, and enabled some essential operations still to be performed. Those patients suffering from cancer were unable to obtain deep radiation and all non-essential operations were cancelled.

The whole country was affected by the power cuts. Electricity Councils appealed to people to reduce the demand for electricity, and a joint statement with the Ministry for the Environment called on Local Authorities to reduce heating and lighting to a minimum compatible with health.

In the exigency of war or natural disaster people try to do their best to cooperate; and even in those lesser circumstances of social unrest most try to help as much as they can. I too was trying to do my best for my obstetric and gynaecological patients for whom I was responsible, for all our non-urgent operations had been cancelled. I was also covering the work of another gynaecologist who was off sick. Looking at her list of operations I noted with amazement that quite a number had been booked for termination of pregnancy. I discussed this problem with Administration and was told that termination of pregnancy was considered to be an emergency and the operation should be performed at all costs, even though it would appear that patients with abnormal bleeding, which might indicate the presence of early cancer, were excluded.

I therefore reviewed the notes of all my colleague's patients who had been booked for legal abortion and noted with increasing disquiet that not one was entitled to termination if the guidance for those requesting termination under the 1967 Abortion Act were correctly observed. What had originally been intended to deal humanely with the occasional patient had now become abortion on demand and the two doctors required by the Act to interview the patients before signing the form of acceptance had cravenly given in to their patients' demands.

I again discussed my anxiety with Administration and was told that we cannot refuse an operation to which the patient has a legal right. I therefore next reviewed the notes of all the patients who had had their operations cancelled and was more than ever concerned to note that some of them had a much greater need for diagnostic appraisal than those for termination that the

Administration had insisted should be operated upon.

I was still young. I needed help. My conscience told me that it was unethical to carry out terminations of pregnancy on some patients while the very lives of others were being put at risk by not having their operations carried out. "What was I to do?" I kept asking myself, "Why did I do medicine? What was my Dream?"

The reading of fairy tales to young children is common to many cultures. All little girls want to be a beautiful princess who needs to be rescued by a brave champion, while every little boy wants to be that champion. Fairy tales, literature, music and movies all borrow from that mythical theme. Sleeping Beauty, Cinderella, Helen of Troy, Romeo and Juliet are such examples. From ancient fables to the latest blockbuster the theme of a strong man coming to rescue a beautiful woman is a deeply felt need of the human psyche. Even the healing profession borrows this deep-seated need of humanity. My dream was to save the life of the suffering and there appeared to be no reason why I should now be asked to take the lives of those who could not defend themselves. Indeed, it made no sense at all! The healthy were to be destroyed and others, who needed life-saving operations, were to be left in abeyance.

The phrase, " between a woman and her physician", which I had fought for was now shown to be an empty one since the physician had now merely become an instrument for carrying out the patient's decision. What about the moral and ethical responsibility of the physician towards his or her patients, and, indeed, what about the physician's observance of the Hippocratic Oath? Yes, I had in my early days seen the complications, which could arise from the ministration of back street abortionists. Indeed, it was those cases that had led me to rebel against the law as it then was. But liberalization of the law had soon degenerated into two doctors acquiescing to the woman's diktat and we were then left with abortion on demand.

After the emergency was over the Government announced

that, due to the cooperation of the medical staff, not one patient in the hospital scene had lost his or her life on account of the emergency measures that had been introduced. However, it failed to take notice of those who had subsequently died due to failure of the system to allow operations for diagnostic purposes to proceed; and I particularly remember one patient who, had she been diagnosed when she should have had her operation, was found six months later to have an inoperable uterine cancer.

Pro- and anti-abortion groups are both vociferous in attempting to get their message across but, in reality, they have little idea of what goes on in practice.

The pro-abortion lobby was the first to become militant. They enlisted the Women's Movement and Broad Churchmen in their ranks and used every available device, such as pamphleteering, public demonstrations, exploitation of the media and lobbying of legislative chambers to get their message across. In their early years I was even captivated by their smooth talk. Demonstrations were made outside hospitals and Parliament. Largely as a result of these efforts the Government considered a private member's bill and, as a result, the 1967 Abortion Law was placed on the Statute Book in England where I was training. Soon however, as is now well known, what was intended to help an occasional tragic case came to be regarded as the norm, and we were, and still are, left with abortion on demand.

Being told that it was my duty to carry out abortions, whatever the justification, was the last straw. This uncompromising order was issued to doctors in hospitals throughout the country and led to some gynaecologists taking early retirement or emigrating. I also refused, and it was the main, if not the only reason, that persuaded my husband and me to leave Britain for a country where abortion, at that time, was rarely practised.

Frozen Pelvis

Margaret, aged 37, attended my consulting rooms in a very disturbed state of mind to enquire whether laser surgery would enable her to conceive. She had been attending doctors for fifteen years, sometimes relying on the National Health Service, and, when she had money, seeing specialists privately, in an effort to obtain help to achieve a pregnancy.

When she was 20 years old she underwent termination of pregnancy at the 10th week. Two years later she had an ectopic pregnancy (a pregnancy occurring in a part of the body other than in the uterine cavity). The gynaecologist who dealt with it reported the presence of numerous pelvic adhesions (where parts of the body stick together, usually as the result of trauma or infection). He treated her conservatively, at the patient's request, by milking out the pregnancy from the right Fallopian tube. A year later, since she had not conceived, he re-laparoscoped her and found what was essentially a frozen pelvis (a condition in which all the pelvic organs are adherent). Since that time she had seen many doctors, and had even changed her life long partner, without being able to achieve her longed for pregnancy. Latterly, besides the lower abdominal discomfort from which she had always suffered since her tubal pregnancy, she had begun to suffer from hot flushes. Hormonal investigations indicated that she had developed a premature menopause. In view of this she underwent in vitro fertilization with egg donation, again without success.

I was very concerned about her, for all her youth and, indeed, her finances, too, had been expended in trying to become pregnant. She wanted me to tell her why she had had an ectopic pregnancy, why she had a frozen pelvis, why an early menopause, and why even egg donation had failed.

I asked her what answers the other doctors had given her. She gazed at the floor and, after a sigh, told me, "I don't think that any of them gave me an answer." I asked her if she had any thoughts about it herself. She replied, "I only know I have not been the same since the abortion."

I was sad that, in spite of all our modern day skills with laser and In Vitro Fertilization, we are still so often unable to help our patients. Truly, in this case at least, and almost certainly in many others, a Pandora's Box is opened when one undergoes termination of pregnancy. It is, of course, well known that pelvic infection may follow this procedure, but why should I.V.F. fail? I had several years before had the honour to work with Dr Patrick Steptoe, the father of I.V.F., and in my own case records had noted that I.V.F. failed more often in those patients who had had a termination of pregnancy in the past than in other patients so treated. Unfortunately, to date, no research has been undertaken in this context. However, it seems likely to me that the termination may damage the endometrium (the lining cells of the uterus) to a lesser extent than that which would produce an Asherman's Syndrome, but, nevertheless, sufficiently to prevent implantation. For those unfamiliar with Asherman's Syndrome they are referred to the case history of that name where they will find that all is revealed.

Animal Lover

Lucy, a woman of 35, visited my clinic in a sombre and somewhat thoughtful frame of mind. She had had two children who had finally started school and so she, at long last, had some spare time to devote to the welfare of animals. This had been her overriding passion for many years. As a child she had owned a pony but had spent so much of her time with it that her parents, noting that her schooling was suffering, made her sell it. Nevertheless, she continued to ride at some nearby stables where, when not riding, she devoted much of her spare time in helping out, and at the same time, became involved with the Royal Society for the Prevention of Cruelty to Animals.

She was very upset at hearing about the poor quality of animal care in many zoological gardens and circuses, but, when she read a newspaper report that pregnant mares were being kept solely by a pharmaceutical company to produce pregnant mares' serum for use in one of their drugs, she became so angry that she decided to devote the rest of her life to the welfare of animals. The finding, therefore, that she was six weeks pregnant came as a terrible shock. She requested termination of pregnancy, and tubal ligation (tying off of uterine tubes to prevent descent of ovum, ascent of spermatozoa, and consequently. the inability to conceive).

I was able to confirm by ultrasound that she was pregnant and thought it wise, therefore, to find out a little more about her overriding passion. I started talking to her about animals, for we were both animal lovers and I had lived on a farm during my childhood years. We told each other about sick animals and abandoned baby animals, and I praised her for being concerned with the weak that could not voice their feelings.

I said that we must be grateful to Richard Martin M.P, who piloted the first anti-cruelty bill through Parliament in 1822 which gave a modicum of protection to cattle, horses and sheep. In 1824 the Royal Society for the Prevention of Cruelty to Animals was founded, the first society in the world to afford protection to animals. Lucy replied that most of the other people who had supported animal rights had been women!

It seemed extraordinary to me that such a sensitive woman, where animals were concerned, could with equanimity, consider terminating her own child and not consider that such a procedure might have long term psychological consequences. The fact that on rare occasions an animal rejects her offspring suggested to me that if I could understand that phenomenon, then I might be the more able to comprehend such human reasoning.

We talked about animals in the wild and also in captivity and the psychological effects of stress. She said that she had read a paper which said that apes never abandon or reject their young, however diseased or crippled the baby may be. However, she also said that the females of several classes of mammals, including lions, mice and certain types of monkey, will either spontaneously abort their foetuses or abandon their newborn when difficulties arise, and she herself had cared for abandoned animals. She was looking forward to the day when animal welfare was paramount and animal cruelty was no more. She herself intended to undertake a political campaign to persuade the government to pass legislation so that her vision could be achieved.

I, on the other hand, was thinking how complex animal behaviour and also human behaviour is. Some things depend on the genetic programme (DNA) in the animal. Others are dependent on the environment in which the embryo develops, and also its subsequent growth to adulthood. Even the cosmos may influence the developing foetus or child e.g. seasonal disease, miscarriage, winter depression. We examined these things and briefly undertook a philosophical discussion as to why a mother might reject her baby, or even her unborn child.

Finally we agreed that, although her reasoning was understandable, nevertheless, further thought was needed, and I made another appointment for her to see me with her husband, in a week's time. During that period she analysed her thoughts and finally decided to keep the pregnancy going. Whether our somewhat lengthy discussion was responsible for her change of mind, or whether the extra time enabled her to adjust more to her new pregnancy state it is difficult to say, but whatever the cause, she started to look forward to the birth of her new baby, whom she subsequently loved dearly.

With the arrival of a new baby her desire to influence the national appreciation of animal welfare naturally required modification, but she maintained her interest by accommodating stray and maltreated animals. Obviously this voluntary work, as well as the care of a young baby, occupied all her time.

Denial

Vanessa was a 38-year-old Information Technologist married to a diplomat, who appeared to be having a vivid and exciting dream of her recent childbirth. There was music and dancing. She was the centre of joyful attention and everyone was congratulating her. She awoke, but she could still hear the music, loud and clear. "I must be dreaming", she thought. She heard the anaesthetic nurse saying, "Open your eyes". She stretched out her hand to fondle her baby, but could not find her. She felt her abdomen but she was not pregnant. She heard the nurse again calling, "It's all over, Vanessa, You're in the Recovery Room".

She opened her eyes. She could not hear music any more. There was no party. She was all alone with only the nurse to attend to her. She suddenly burst into tears and screamed, "I want my baby! Please do not take my baby away," She continued to scream, and she made so much noise that I could hear her in the adjoining theatre where I was operating laparoscopically with laser on a patient with massive pelvic endometriosis (the presence of cells from the lining of the uterus in abnormal positions) which needed all my concentration. I knew that the hospital did not have a maternity unit and wondered therefore why a patient was asking for her baby.

After I had finished the operation I accompanied my patient to the Recovery Room and there saw the patient whom I had heard. She was still violently sobbing, in spite of having been given strong sedation. I felt very sorry for her at that moment. No one could comfort her because she was still under the influence of the anaesthetic and not properly awake; or was she awake and had just woken up to the reality of the situation?

I saw Vanessa six weeks later at the request of her gynaecologist who had gone away on holiday. To my relief she was a quite different lady to the one whom I had seen in the Recovery Room six weeks previously. She was very chic, well dressed and made up, and was getting ready to accompany her husband to an overseas diplomatic posting. Although I had seen her and knew a little of her story, she had never seen me before.

I glanced at her notes and asked how she was feeling. She replied stiffly and without a smile that she was very well, and appeared to be in a hurry to get the interview and examination over as quickly as possible. I said, "Do you have any problems?" She gave a brief, supercilious smile, as if to imply, "What a strange question", and said, "Of course I have no problems." I persisted and said, "What about emotional problems?" She replied, "Certainly not. Why should I have emotional problems? The termination was of my own choosing." I was dumbfounded. I appeared to be speaking to an entirely different person to the one I had seen, barely six weeks previously, in a state of abject distress. I hesitatingly continued, "But you were very distressed after your operation. No one could calm you." She flared up at my persistence and angrily denied that she had been in any way disturbed by the operation.

The rest of the meeting and examination was almost conducted in silence. I marvelled that an intelligent woman who had been so distraught by the result of the operation six weeks previously, and had pleaded with the nursing staff for help, was so quickly able to erect an iron curtain around herself and, apparently, to block out all memory of her waking moments. Did she really have no remembrance of her extreme distress, or was this a brave façade that she had erected to fool herself and others? Did she feel anger, shame, isolation, and had attempted to resolve her emotional conflict by self-denial, or had she really no remembrance of that day? I decided that I would discuss the problem with our psychiatrist.

He said that it was not only some patients who deny the abortion but all of us deny what is happening. The silent majority look around and do not want to think about it because it is so depressing. They just want to get on with their own lives, while, all the time, 500 babies are being aborted each day in the United Kingdom, carried out in their hospitals, funded by their taxes and performed on their neighbours or friends. While the mothers, who are destroying their own babies, remain silent, as they think they must, then society will continue to deny and ignore their pain. In one way or another we are all like this lady and deny it!

Unexplained Itch

Mary, a 36-year-old Irish Australian, arrived in my Sydney consulting rooms in an old, lace-fringed dress of a bygone age. She was certainly not slim but her slovenly appearance suggested that her will to look smart had eventually failed and that she had finally given up the unequal struggle. It was a late autumn day and the afternoon sun, which was shining through the consulting room window, outlined the blemishes in her attire. She handed me the questionnaire that all my patients were requested to fill in before they saw me and took the seat that I offered her. She looked disconsolate, even battered, and one could tell that she had had a hard life.

I glanced at the questionnaire to give her time to collect her thoughts, and she began to say, "I hope you can help me. I've had this itch down below for many years. I've seen many doctors and have used many medicines. I've even had a hysterectomy (surgical removal of the uterus), but nothing has helped." She had had four children and a termination. Nothing else in her history appeared to be relevant.

Examination was also unrewarding. She had a scar in her abdomen, the consequence of her hysterectomy, but that was all. Even the pelvic examination failed to reveal any inflammation that might suggest an infection, and the vulval skin also appeared to be healthy. What could explain her condition? I inspected the entire area with the colposcope, which is a type of microscope for examining the lower genital tract. I took some swabs and some blood for investigation, and I even took a biopsy of the area that she pointed out to me, and arranged to see her during the following week.

When she next came I explained that none of the tests that I had taken had shown any sign of infection nor, indeed, any abnormality at all. I tried to reassure her. Then, as an after thought, she said, "Doctor, could it be the result of the termination?" She went on to explain that the problem had started shortly after she had had the termination ten years previously. She said, "Doctor, sometimes the itch is so bad that I want to have the whole area cut out." It seemed improbable that a hysterectomy had been performed on account of the pruritus (itch) from which she suffered so I asked again why she had had a hysterectomy and she again replied that it was because of the vulval itch.

It occurred to me that she might well have been right that the induced abortion had something to do with the miserable state that she now found herself in, so I questioned her about her view on termination of pregnancy. She said, "Doctor, I am a Catholic and what I have done is against the teaching of the church. As I am really not a religious person I thought it would not affect me. Since I came to Australia I have been involved in biology and a certain amount of animal research, and now I realize that life really does start from a single fertilized cell. Then I ask myself, 'How could I have destroyed it?'"

She continued, "When I attended the doctor I was two weeks overdue. He rushed me to hospital and, after the curettage to procure the abortion, he told me that there was really nothing there. Looking back now I realize that if there was nothing there then what was the rush. Was it all just a fairy story? Now I have woken up to reality. It's now too late. I know now that that little thing, no bigger than a grain of sugar, was all that was needed. Nothing else had to be added. We all began life as a single cell!" She could have gone on for an hour lecturing me about biology, and how human life began.

I showed interest in her research and encouraged her to write a book about her findings. In reality, I thought Mary resented her genitalia on account of feelings of guilt and wanted to punish herself by removing everything connected with her sin. "Do you," I asked, "wash yourself there frequently?" She confessed that she was washing down below nearly all the time.

I suggested that it might be helpful if she saw a counsellor, or possibly a psychiatrist, but she replied that she had seen many different doctors. She was convinced that she had some gynaecological problem and she wanted me to help her to achieve a cure. Her apparent faith in me was extremely disconcerting. I myself was persuaded that there was no undiscovered pathology to account for her pruritus or irritation, but how was I to convince Mary of that fact?

I started by telling her to stop all medications, even soap, not to have more than one shower a day, and I repeated my investigations, even going to the length of taking a vulval biopsy. As I suspected, all investigations drew a blank. At a further consultation I discussed with her all the known causes of vulval itch, or pruritus vulvae as it is called by the medical profession. I told her to avoid using bubble baths and explained that allergies could sometimes be responsible, as indeed could excessive washing. I discussed the two most common causes of vulval itch, the fungal infection, candidiasis, and the, nowadays, less common protozoan infection, trichomoniasis, and explained that the swabs that I had taken had excluded those infections, as well as the miscellaneous bacterial organisms that could be responsible for bacterial vaginosis. In any case, clinical examination had already indicated that such conditions were unlikely to be present. Finally, the vulval biopsy had been able to totally exclude more exotic skin conditions, such as lichen sclerosus or psoriasis.

After a further three visits I was able to persuade Mary that there was no pathology that required treatment. The hysterectomy, it appeared, had been entirely unnecessary, and had been performed, at her insistence, to get rid of the itch.

Mary, I gathered, had led a fairly restricted childhood, and any wrongdoing was considered to be a sin for which she needed absolution from the local priest. "We all have a built in conscience," I explained to Mary, "which tells us when we are doing wrong, and this is what is goading you." Mary agreed and said that a feeling of guilt over the long-passed termination was still nagging her. Surprisingly, the more she became familiar with biology the more her feelings of guilt plagued her. We jointly came to the conclusion that her guilty feelings were the cause of her illness; and she said that she now understood that she needed to be sorted out, because the unwanted pregnancy and the painful experience of the subsequent abortion, although they occurred so many years ago, still tore at her soul. We finally agreed that we would both write something about her experience and she accepted my advice that she should consult a counsellor, and that she would also get involved in any way she could to offer help to others who might have had similar experiences.

When I saw her a year later she had fully accepted the fact that her symptom was psychosomatic and, more importantly, had discovered that she was not alone. She had joined a therapy group which enabled its members to share their often similar, sad stories and obtain strength from the shared knowledge.

IVF and its Dilemma

I have combined two peoples' stories in the following passage because, although one of their histories was not associated with an abortion episode, they were so inextricably linked in my mind with similar medical problems that they are better treated together.

I must first of all say a little about In Vitro Fertilization (IVF). All professionals, if they are worth their salt, seek perfection, The tennis player trains five hours a day to perfect his skills, the ballerina does likewise to perfect her balance, while even the priest is for ever examining his conscience.

The Obstetrician, who continues to hone his or her skills by practical experience, by reading medical journals, and by attending medical meetings and congresses from the time of graduation to the time of retirement has, as the objective, the safe delivery of a healthy baby to a healthy mother. In the past awareness for the mother began with quickening, although she might suspect that she was pregnant by the cessation of her periods or the development of amenorrhoea as it is usually termed . The Obstetrician, too, really only became concerned about the baby's welfare when the foetal heart could be heard with the Pinard stethoscope; although bimanual examination might suggest that the patient was pregnant at a much earlier date.

Nowadays we are involved with the baby from fertilization. We study the baby, we see it with 3 D or 4 D Ultrasound, and we hear its heart beat with Doppler. We see the baby's every movement. We see it sucking its thumb. We see its reaction to music. We see its multiple emotions, and Dr Bernard N. Nathanson, who at one time was the director of the largest abortion clinic in the world, having witnessed, by means of ultrasound, the anguish of a foetus being aborted, became one of the leading lights in the fight to protect those tiniest of mortals. Not only may we see and hear the foetus, but we can nowadays treat him in utero for certain conditions, and we have to thank the late Professor Albert William Liley in New Zealand for his pioneering work in this regard.

Some years ago I joined an In Vitro Fertilization Centre in London where I had the honour of working with Dr Patrick Steptoe, the father of I.V.F.. Every year millions of couples try to conceive, but many are unsuccessful, and, in some cases, no cause is found. Dr Steptoe, a Gynaecologist in Oldham General Hospital, and Dr Robert Edwards, a physiologist in Cambridge University, UK, worked from 1966 for ten years to try to find a solution to the problem and in 1977 the first I.V.F. baby was born, an event that shook the scientific world to its foundations.

Since that day thousands of clinicians and scientists have worked hard to help infertile couples to achieve the longed for pregnancy that they have not managed to obtain by any other means. Those patients who attend I.V.F. Centres require a certain amount of bravery to endure the discomfort of many of the procedures to which they are subjected and, more importantly, to tolerate the embarrassment which may occur when their personal and private lives are discussed by the hospital staff who are attempting to help them.

Egg collection is an anxious time for all concerned. The gynaecologist collects the eggs, usually trans-vaginally with a long needle, under ultrasound control, from the hyper-stimulated ovaries. The nurse hastens to deliver them to the embryologist, and another nurse also rushes the partner's prepared semen to the same embryologist who incubates them in a medium that mimics the fluid in the uterine tubes. On the following day the embryologist, if some of the eggs have been fertilized, appears at the door like a conquering knight to report the good news to all the I.V.F. staff and to the patient herself. There is general rejoicing, or, in case of failure, a feeling of sadness or disappointment. In the former case the gynaecologist, and the patient too, are invited to look down the microscope and see the beginnings of life. One sees two cells that may divide as one observes the miracle and that one hopes will, in some 270 days, issue forth into the full light of day as a new born baby.

My object in this lengthy preamble is to introduce you to two patients who were fertilized and became pregnant on the same day and who, a little later, formed the bulk of our discussion in one of the weekly meetings in the department.

The first patient, Fereste's husband, was a young man of 22, in the prime of life, who, in the course of war, had both his legs and buttocks blown away and his vasa deferentia (a portion of the excretory system of the testis down which the spermatozoa pass) severed. He took off his eternity ring and sent it back to Fereste, together with a photograph of himself as he then was, and a letter explaining the situation and saying, "I cannot marry you. Now I am a different person." Fereste joined him in the hospital, insisted on marrying him and, two years later, he saw me in the hospital in his wheel chair and told me his history with much emotion. He told me that he had lost everything but he did not want to lose his wife as well, whom he loved so very much.

Examination and investigations revealed that he had azoospermia i.e. the absence of live spermatozoa in the semen due, it was thought, to the injuries that he had sustained, and which was irreversible. I arranged for our urologist to see him and it was decided that the only chance of success would be if sperm retrieval, using a micro-surgical method, were employed. Micro-epididymal sperm aspiration was therefore scheduled to take place at the same time that Fereste's eggs were due to be collected (the epididymis is that portion of the seminal duct where the spermatozoa are at first stored after they have been made in the testis). Some of the semen was inseminated with the eggs and intra-cyto-plasmic sperm injection was also employed at the same time. The latter procedure had only just been perfected. Essentially, a single retrieved sperm was micro-injected into one of the wife's eggs and after the third attempt success was achieved. No doubt, the fact that the couple were young and basically healthy was helpful. The romantic love story was known to many of the I.V.F. staff and there was general rejoicing which reached its acme when a positive pregnancy test was announced.

About a month later when the I.V.F. Unit held one of its weekly meeting to discuss the successes and failures that had occurred, the case just described was placed at the top of the agenda. The second case that was debated was of quite a different nature. Another couple who had had three attempts to achieve a pregnancy, but without success, ended by selling their home so that they could have a final attempt. Three embryos were transferred on the same day as the micro-injection of Fereste's egg was found to have been fertilized. Pregnancy testing confirmed that the latter patient, Lucy, had also become pregnant. Three embryos had been inserted, two survived and ultrasound confirmed that she had twins. Instead of joy at the announcement Lucy became extremely angry and unhappy. She maintained that she only wanted one baby and demanded termination. She did, however, grudgingly agree that she would consider elective foetal reduction and selective termination.

The sunshine that had been lighting up the department for several weeks was suddenly obscured by the dark cloud of discontent generated by Lucy's demand for termination. The rest of the meeting was spent in discussing the management of multiple pregnancy. We had been in the habit of transferring three embryos with the hope that at least one would survive. It was decided that in future only two embryos would be transferred. Our aim was to achieve a pregnancy that resulted in a live birth with one or more infants and with minimal neonatal mortality and morbidity. Some of the team agreed that selective termination was acceptable in cases of foetal abnormality, especially when the lives of all the foetuses were at risk, but no one thought that there was any indication for selective termination in Lucy's case.

Sadly, Lucy attended another gynaecologist in another hospital who agreed to her request. The operation was performed and one of the twins was aborted. The remaining twin subsequently aborted spontaneously.

The announcement that a British gynaecologist had selectively reduced a twin pregnancy to a single one for social reasons soon became widely known. It was reported by the press on both sides of the Atlantic and caused quite a furore. I was unable to understand the philosophy, either behind the wife's request, or of the gynaecologist's reasoning. Are we medical practitioners technicians, without feelings or consciences, who are obliged to obey the dictate of our patients, to build up or to destroy, purely as they demand?

Shatterd World of a Man

Miss C came to see me requesting termination of pregnancy. After the consultation I suggested that I should speak to her boy friend, George, since, as I was at pains to explain, there were three people to consider. This I did and her boy friend made it very clear to me that he was very opposed to the suggestion that the pregnancy should be terminated. They had been living together for quite some time and had not used contraception, so the conclusion that he had reached was that a pregnancy would be welcome.

I called in Miss C and told her what her partner had said. Miss C had fully decided to have an abortion. Indeed, her mind was closed to any thought of an alternative, and any rational discussion was quite impossible. George, in the meantime, was very disturbed. He kept walking backwards and forwards, running out to the car, chain smoking, and all the time, beads of sweat were forming on his forehead and cheekbones and running down. He begged his partner, "Please keep our baby." He continued, "I love you, and this is the fruit of our love. This is our baby!"

It appeared that they had discussed the pregnancy before they saw me, but Miss C had erected a powerful barrier, impervious to any rational appeal of her partner, and deaf to anything that I might say. She was wealthy. Her career would suffer if she had a baby, and in any case, why should she share her wealth with her boy friend if he became the father of her child? This, indeed, she was honest enough to tell me when I saw her alone.

Since the fruit of procreation usually arises from the consent of two people it seemed to me that any decision about the welfare of the unborn child should be made by the agreement of both parents. This heartless and heart-rending scene played out before me put me in mind of a similar case played out in the High Court of Parliament in 1987 when an Oxford University student made a last-ditch plea for the life of his unborn love child. He lost his battle. It appears that in the United Kingdom, and also in the United States, a father has no authority by law to prohibit the mother of his child from terminating a pregnancy. The decision rests solely with the woman, provided she can convince two doctors that she meets the criteria laid out under the 1967 Abortion Act as amended by the 1990 Human Fertilisation and Embryology Act. On the other hand a man can make a girl pregnant and then take no further responsibility for her or for the child. Truly, the Law is incongruous. It should be noted that in many parts of the world the exact opposite prevails, and all children's rights devolve to the father. This is an equally unsatisfactory state of affairs.

George continued, "I will help and protect you. If you have an abortion I shall never know in this life if my child was a boy or a girl. I find it almost impossible to know why you want to do away with it."

A week later George phoned me to say that his partner had had an abortion. She continued to bleed heavily and was very upset. In anguish George said, "How could I comfort her when she, herself, had made the decision?" They parted in acrimony.

Alleged Rape

Chantelle, a young girl of fourteen, was brought to my Consulting Rooms in Sydney, Australia, by her mother who requested that I should terminate her pregnancy. The mother told me that she had become pregnant because her bedroom window had been left open and someone must have climbed in and made her pregnant without her being aware of the fact!

Chantelle remained silent when I questioned her and obviously did not wish to answer my questions while her mother was present. Since this was a serious matter that might involve rape of a minor, and the possibility of venereal infection, I asked the mother to wait outside for a few minutes while I examined her and asked her further questions.

Although poorly educated, Chantelle was nevertheless intelligent and she immediately commenced to answer my questions in a mature and truthful manner. Her family were poor and her father had left them when she was only four, so her mother had a hard job to make ends meet. She was disgruntled and rarely spoke to Chantelle except to criticize her. There did not appear to be much affection shared between the two and Chantelle's one joy was a broken doll that had been given to her.

For the past year or so she had been acutely aware of her increasing height and her rapid development into womanhood.

She hated school and looked forward to the time when she would become a mother and have her own home, for she realized that, however old she became, she would forever remain a child while she lived with her mother. Sadly, Chantelle was never able to discuss with her mother any of the things that really mattered to her.

Having given her free range to describe her family life, I asked her if she had a boyfriend. She told me that she had had a steady boyfriend for more than a year and a half, whom she loved dearly and who returned her love. How wonderful it would be, she said, to live with him in their own home and to look after a growing family. She just wanted to have her own live doll that no one could ever take from her. Other possessions did not interest her.

I then asked her why she thought she was pregnant. Chantelle said that for the last two years her periods had been regular but that she had missed the last two and therefore thought she might be pregnant. She would go to the nearby bush and try to decide if she should tell her mother, who would be frightfully angry, especially as she had warned her against her growing attachment to the youth, and had said that if she did fall pregnant he would probably be sent to prison. When she finally plucked up courage to speak to her mother she discovered that she was not as angry as she had feared, but had insisted that if the pregnancy was confirmed it must be terminated.

Chantelle confessed that she could not sleep the night before she saw me, for not only did she fear for the safety of her boyfriend but also she could not face the prospect that her pregnancy might be terminated.

I asked Chantelle to tell me more about her boyfriend. She pursed her full, thick lips and grinned as she thought of their blossoming relationship. She brightened momentarily, but then became more sober and replied, "I love my boyfriend. He's the only one I've got. But, please, doctor, I'm frightened." Her long lashed eyes widened with apprehension. I smiled and said, "Don't be afraid." By this time Chantelle's eyes were swimming with tears. She stopped a big tear from falling with the back of her hand. I attempted to sooth her and said, "No one's going to hurt you here." She then asked in a frightened whisper, "Are you going to take my baby from me?" "Of course not," I replied, "but let's first see if you are pregnant." Pelvic examination and ultrasound both confirmed that she was indeed just over eight weeks pregnant, and the latter demonstrated the presence of a healthy heart beat. I was also pleased to note that there was no evidence of pelvic or venereal infection.

I saw the mother again, confirmed that Chantelle was pregnant, and, in order to avoid a possibly unpleasant altercation with her, said that Chantelle should be seen by a social worker. Since I also was fairly new to Sydney, I discussed with our lawyer the characteristics of the Abortion Law in New South Wales and the social rights of that young girl. He told me that although Australian Law was based on British Law, nevertheless, the law concerning Abortion was different in each of the States. The Royal Commission on Human Relationships in 1977 had reported that 60,000 abortions were carried out in Australia during the previous year.

In New South Wales various counselling services were available: Social Services, as well as various Churches and Pro-life Organizations were there to advise, as well as Legal Aid and certain Voluntary Agencies; while numerous Abortion Clinics had also sprung up.

Suffice it to say that arrangements were made for Chantelle to be cared for. Eventually she and her boyfriend were married. Social Services made housing available for them, and her mother was pacified. Chantelle became an almost regular visitor to my Consulting Rooms. She was always simply dressed but most of her care was lavished on the baby who was immaculately turned out. A second baby was soon on the way, and when I left Australia some seven or eight years later she was the proud mother of four young children.

Although it is clear that this did not turn out to be a case of rape it provides a suitable place for this important topic to be aired, particularly as it is frequently made an excuse for termination of pregnancy, and indeed, because it was a major factor in persuading the United Kingdom government to introduce the Abortion Act in 1967.

It is certainly true that a woman's request for abortion, following rape, is a cry for help, but how often, in fact, does rape lead to pregnancy? A woman is only capable of being fertilized for about three days during her thirty-day cycle and, in the case of rape, psychological and physiological factors also play an important part in limiting the risk of a resulting pregnancy. It has been estimated that the chance of becoming pregnant after one episode of unprotected sexual intercourse is about 5%.

This is not to say that rape is not dreadfully traumatic for the victim. Indeed, it must be one of the most distressing experiences that any woman can face. It is a problem that has beset society for millennia. It is almost certainly under-reported, due most likely, to fear of retaliation by the perpetrator of the crime, and also for fear of public humiliation. Incidentally, it would seem that rapists usually commit their crimes for the feeling of power that they wield over their victim, rather than for sexual gratification.

Victims of rape need supportive care without delay if they are not to suffer, not only immediate, but often life-long effects. The former will include unpredictable and intense emotions, jumpiness, flash-backs, sleeplessness, nightmares, and lack of concentration; while long term psychological effects will not only include all the former symptoms, but may in addition lead to self-harm and self-blame. Early psychological and, often, psychiatric help for these people is therefore essential.

Male rape is also becoming more recognized, and has certainly become commoner since same-sex relationships were permitted by the governments of many countries. The effects of such abuse are likely to be even more calamitous than for female victims because of the sense of shame that is engendered and the consequent disinclination to seek help. Appropriate psychological and psychiatric aid is, therefore, all the more necessary.

Incest is also not uncommon, and is certainly under-reported. The victim may suffer the same symptoms as the person who has been raped. An incidence of between 2 and 4% in close family members has been reported. Although abuse by stepfathers has been most commonly described, nevertheless, fathers have also been incriminated. However, it is generally believed that the most common form of incest occurs between brothers and sisters.

Obtaining statistics of rape in different countries is difficult, and results quoted, even of the same year, can differ wildly. The 2005 National Crime Victimization Study in America said that 64,080 women were raped in 2004. However, another study for the same year put the figure at 200,780! In England and Wales a Home Office Study, also for 2004, indicated that 190,000 serious assaults occurred against women in England and Wales, of which 80,000 were rape, or attempted rape. However, those men charged because of the Sexual Offences Act numbered only 13,322. South Africa and the Seychelles are said to have the highest incidence of rape in the world with Australia coming third. Possibly this is because the victims are more willing to report the crime.

Obviously rape increases exponentially in War, as has been made obvious from reports emanating from the Congo and Darfur. Statistics from third world countries are usually either scanty or absent. Muslim countries, but certainly not the Sudan, would appear to have very low numbers of rapes, but is that really so? In Pakistan a legal activist, Uzma Saeed, is campaigning on behalf of women for the repeal of the controversial Hudood Laws which rule that all extra-marital sex is illegal; for she has shown that those laws are completely manipulated by the men. Thus, if a woman alleges that she has been raped, she has to provide four pious male witnesses or face a charge of adultery! How on earth can she do that? In other words, it allows Pakistani men to rape with impunity.

As far as my own experience is concerned I have, in 37 years of medical practice, come across only one case of incest and one case of rape where the victims have become pregnant. This tends to confirm the belief that psychological and physiological factors also contribute to the low pregnancy rate following rape.

Gender Selection

Sunita, a 28-year-old Indian lady domiciled in the United Kingdom, came to see me requesting amniocentesis to determine the sex of her unborn child. I had expected to see a demure, shy person, dressed in an exquisite, brightly coloured sari, for she was immensely rich, but I found instead a sophisticated and Anglicized young lady attired in a smart trouser suit. She had, it would seem, entirely abandoned her Indian culture in exchange for a supercilious, Western approach. Strangely enough I was soon to discover that she had not abandoned the philosophy and thought processes that she had inherited. I asked if there was a gender-related illness in the family. She smiled and replied, "This is my third pregnancy. I have two daughters and would like a son. I just couldn't face having another daughter". This request came in such a natural way as to make me suppose that she thought I fully understood how important gender selection was for her.

As I always try to help my patients, both medically and psychologically if I ethically can, I attempted to discover something about her appreciation of the dilemma as it impinged upon her ethical and religious beliefs. She said that she was a Hindu and believed in reincarnation. She was also a vegetarian and did not eat meat because it involved taking animal life which she held to be sacred. She finally expressed the view that there was no law against abortion in Hinduism.

I suggested that she could have an amniocentesis for health reasons, but not purely for sex determination. She left my clinic unhappily, presumably to buy her desire from an abortion clinic.

It is interesting to note that during the same month six other Indian patients attended my consulting rooms with similar requests. Their stories were all somewhat alike, and I have chosen just one as an illustration. With all these patients I was faced with a similar dilemma, for I wanted to help them if I could. The year before I had travelled extensively in India and had taken the opportunity to discuss the question of abortion with one of their priests who was also medically qualified.

Hindu medical ethics, it would seem, is based on the principle of 'ahimsa' or non-violence, and is therefore opposed to abortion, unless it is to save the mother's life; similar, in fact, to what it was in the West before abortion became liberalized. Besides having seen cows wandering around the streets, especially in Varanasi, and sometimes defrauding store holders of their produce, I remembered visiting a Jain temple on Malabar Hill in Bombay where the priests and other occupants were wearing masks over their noses so that they did not, inadvertently, damage or kill any insects with which they might come in contact. In view of this basic philosophy of non-violence it is surprising that female foeticide is so readily carried out. It would seem too, that the practice of suttee, the action of self-immolation of the wife on her late husband's funeral pyre, has still not been completely eliminated. How strange that Indian womanhood, that has been seeking for millennia for sexual equality, should so lightly esteem the gift of female life.

According to the doctrine of reincarnation the soul inhabits the embryo from conception, and therefore killing the embryo or foetus has a deleterious effect on its 'karma' or fate. Indeed, even the Indian Government in 1996 placed a ban on sex-selection. All the Hindu Scriptures condemn abortion and are therefore at one with Judaism, Christianity and Islam in censuring this operation.

This, and similar cases with which I had to deal, made me search the literature to discover something of the culture and beliefs of the many patients from India and the Far East who were my patients. Although their religion condemned abortion, nevertheless, once their religious tenets had been sidestepped, termination of pregnancy became no more of a problem to most people in the East than it has become for many in the Western world.

Female selective abortion is most common in countries, such as India, where a large dowry must be paid on marriage. Many poor peasant families are quite unable to cope with the large dowry expected by the family into which their daughter is to marry and consequently prefer not to run the risk of having a daughter at all. There is also the belief by some Indians that female children are less worthy than their male counterparts because they leave home and family when they marry. A further factor is the fear that their daughter, when married, may suffer the fate of 'dowry death' in which the bride is either murdered by the groom's family or commits suicide because of abuse or neglect. It is shocking to read that about 7,000 'dowry deaths' were reported to have taken place in India in 2003.

Male selective abortion is rare, for sons are more likely than daughters to provide farm labour, or to enter the family business, and to support their parents when they are old. Sons are also needed to continue the family line and eventually to kindle their parent's funeral pyre and to assist in the salvation of their souls.

Gender selection is not confined to India. It is practised in many countries in the Far East, including China, South Korea and Taiwan. It probably accounts for the fact that males outnumber females in those countries, despite the fact that males have a higher death rate than females.

It should be pointed out that female selective abortion is not the only means by which unwanted females are destroyed. Indians, like the Chinese, also resort to postnatal infanticide. The parents sometimes approach the traditional midwife or Dais, as she is called, to aid them in their request. Immediately after birth, if the newborn child is a baby girl, the midwife is induced to suddenly and roughly invert the child, thereby snapping her spinal cord. The baby is then declared to be stillborn. This, of course, was the normal method by which baby girls were disposed of in the days before intrauterine sex determination enabled the foetus to be destroyed in utero.

In an attempt to outlaw this custom, Indian laboratories are forbidden by law to reveal the foetus's sex that has been discovered by ultrasound scan or amniocentesis. Needless to say not all laboratories obey the rule. Indeed, it was recently reported in 'The Lancet' that more than ten million female foetuses were aborted in India during the previous twenty years.

In the United States, and some of the more prosperous and technologically advanced Western nations, pre-pregnancy sex selection methods are now being commercially encouraged by the Assisted Reproduction industry. Sperms can now be sorted; the woman chooses the sex that she wants and, for an expensive fee, the sperm likely to fulfil her desire is then implanted into her egg! The risks of treating children as commodities rather than as God given human beings, of changing sex ratios in local populations, and of further commercializing reproduction are only too obvious.

People in the West tend to be shocked by female selective abortion and by post-natal infanticide as practised in India, China and other countries in the Far East. What hypocrisy! The abuses of pre-pregnancy sex selection there are just as great, and if they carry on as they are going, it will not be long before infanticide becomes acceptable. Sunita, of course, was not dissuaded from having a third daughter by lack of money for a future dowry. Rather, she was following fashion and had decided that her third child should be a boy.

The Curse of Infertility

Inoticed the easy grace and erect posture of Sasha as she entered my Consulting Room and took the seat opposite me. Her steady eyes were set wide apart and were framed by long, curling lashes which were accentuated by her arched eyebrows that set off perfectly her exquisitely formed nose and small mouth. The red silk shawl, together with the expensive jewellery that she wore, served to emphasize the gold in her hair. She truly was very beautiful, and must have been the envy of many of her generation. To that was added the fact that she was married to a very wealthy and successful Russian oligarch. What more could she ask for?

I quickly noticed that, in spite of her beauty, a tinge of sadness pervaded her countenance, which I had not at first observed. Her mouth was dry and there was some desperation in the tone of her voice when she said, "Doctor, I want a baby. I've been trying for the last three years without success." She had no other problems, had had no illnesses of note and infertility investigations in her own country had shown no abnormality. She told me that she was very fertile for she had had two terminations when she was 19 and 20 years old. From then onwards she had taken the contraception pill until the age of 34 when she planned to start a family. Now, at 37, she was beginning to get desperate.

She handed me copies of the results of her investigations and

I noticed that neither laparoscopy (inspection of the abdominal cavity with a telescope), nor hysteroscopy (inspection of the uterine cavity with a telescope) had been performed. Those omissions I proceeded to remedy. Hysteroscopic investigation did not reveal any problem but laparoscopic investigation showed that she had thickened tubes with peri-tubal and peri-ovarian adhesions. These I succeeded in separating through the laparoscope with the aid of laser. I then arranged for methylene blue dye to be injected by my assistant through her cervix and was happy to note that the dye passed easily through her uterine tubes into the peritoneal cavity. I finally carried out some hormonal investigations and was glad to note that she appeared to be ovulating.

I did not see Sasha again until eighteen months later. Pregnancy had still not been achieved, so I suggested that assisted conception should be undertaken. Unfortunately, due to her husband's tight work schedule, that undertaking was unduly delayed. Eventually In Vitro Fertilization was performed in Russia, but sadly, all that was achieved was a pelvic infection.

A year later, after that last unfortunate episode, I saw her again in London with her husband. She was pale and drawn, and a look of despair was apparent. Her husband's solemn eyes flickered momentarily with emotion, and his face was flushed. He was really very handsome, and it was obvious that they were both still deeply in love and wanted a pregnancy to bind them even more closely together. To any onlooker it was obvious that they were a perfect couple to have a family, but for them, and more particularly for Sasha, it was a necessity of life.

On this particular occasion it was found that she had a pre-menopausal hormonal profile, and an attempt to stimulate her ovaries failed to produce oocytes. This was like a sentence of death for Sasha, for at one fell swoop, all hope of having a child of her own was taken away.

Sasha was put on hormone replacement therapy, but, although it relieved her of her menopausal symptoms, nevertheless she went into deep depression. To any outsider Sasha appeared to have everything that a Russian woman could want, but for Sasha the one thing that she needed from life had been denied her. She had no baby. The last I heard of Sasha was that she was taking anti-depressants and was still fantasizing about the child that she should have had.

I had a number of Russian patients like Sasha who attended my Consulting Rooms in London, with the hope that I could enable them to become pregnant after they had had failed attempts in Russia. No doubt their quests were encouraged by sympathetic Russian medical colleagues whom I had met at Medical Laser Congresses in St Petersburg or Moscow that I had attended over the years. The plight of these patients encouraged me to make further enquires about fertility and abortion rates in that enormous country of Russia which had only recently been accessible to world-wide scrutiny.

The Soviet Union was the first country in the world to legalize abortion in 1921 in order to proclaim the liberation of women under the Marxist-Leninist banner, and although this law was temporarily suspended during the Second World War, it is still very much in force. According to the Demographic Yearbook of the European Council, and an analogous Demographic Yearbook of the United Nations, Russia is the only country in the world where abortions consistently outnumber live births by a ratio of about 2 to 1. In Russia Maternal Mortality is three times greater than in any other Western country. Early pregnancies, too, often end in abortion. Indeed, abortion, whether spontaneous or induced, remains the main cause of female mortality.

According to Serov, the chief gynaecologist at the Ministry of Health, abortions are the chief cause of infertility in a country which is desperate to raise its falling birth rate. About 13% of Russian married couples are infertile and in almost three out of four cases it is attributable to complications resulting from previous abortions.

Russia's population fell by more than half a million, or 0.3%, in the first eight months of this year and the State Statistics

Committee predict a further decline of 11 million, to about 134 million in the world's largest country by 2015.

The only country in the world that has a higher abortion rate than Russia is Romania. At the present time 3 out of 4 pregnancies are terminated. In a country that has a population of 23 million it is estimated that 800,000 abortions a year are performed!

With these statistics in mind, I thought it might be of interest to revert to Sasha's story and recount her early history as she told it to me over the course of a number of consultations:

Sasha was a student when she first became pregnant. Little family planning was available, and, although she would have liked to have kept the baby, the lack of finance, as well as the lack of space, made such a course of action impracticable. In any case, she was a student, and she would have had to surrender her place at University and forgo her chance of betterment. Besides, the government tended to encourage abortion. She saw the doctor who looked after the students and she arranged for a termination to be carried out, almost as a matter of course.

A year later she became pregnant for the second time. On this occasion she thought long and hard about her condition, but again decided that abortion would be the preferable option. She again saw the student's doctor who scheduled her for an abortion. There was no attempt to counsel her. Afterwards she was sad and had, as she put it, a sickly feeling in her stomach, but that, she was told, was routine. Everyone had to accept it. She was struggling with her emotions but did her best to suppress them. She received no sympathy from any one. Often at that time she suffered from nightmares but did not link them with the underlying cause.

Sasha was an ambitious young lady and, after all, she needed to continue with her education. However, on this occasion, she continued to bleed after the termination for more than a month and experienced discomfort in her pelvic region. She expressed her fears to the doctor who merely said that it was normal. If it was normal, she reasoned, then she had to fight against her growing depression and get on with her life. After all, she had done good service to her country and the world by helping to keep down the population! Later she even forgot that she had had an abortion. One realised, on taking medical histories from Russian patients, that having a termination was considered routine; just like having a cold. It was not considered relevant, and, therefore, unless asked about specifically, was not worth mentioning.

Sasha learnt two foreign languages and became a journalist, a good one at that, and it was while interviewing a very handsome, wealthy and rising star in governmental circles that she met her future husband. He was smitten by her beauty and they married. First they planned to build a large dacha well outside the city limits. No expense was spared. One of the best European architects was chosen and the planning and construction took three years. Marble was brought from Italy and furniture and curtains from Paris.

Sasha told me, before it had become obvious that there was not going to be an heir, that the most important part of the house would be the nursery. There Sasha would be able to bring up her child and, in the evenings if work allowed, her husband would be able to dote on their child who would one day inherit his wealth. She showed me photographs of their dacha that included a long gallery hung with Italian and Russian paintings, and also one of a beautiful lady with an angelic, little three-year-old girl by her side, who she confessed, was herself. She said, at that time to me, "I'm hoping to hang by its side a painting of my own little child. However, the best part of the house will still be the nursery!"

Hydrocephaly

Shirley, aged 24, was a happy, contented girl who was a Naturalist, eating and drinking only natural foods. She bore a hydrocephalic baby (a baby with a large head due to an increased amount of cerebo-spinal fluid within the skull) in her second pregnancy. Shirley's first child was 10 months old when she became pregnant again. She was still breast-feeding and the pregnancy was unexpected.

On examination, Shirley was found to be 22 weeks pregnant. She was very surprised and shocked at the news. Ultrasound was carried out and this demonstrated foetal heartbeat and foetal movements. This delighted Shirley and from then on she was very happy about the pregnancy. A repeat ultrasound at the 28th week however was suspicious of hydrocephaly. The situation was explained, genetic counselling was carried out and serial ultrasound scans were thereafter performed. Eventually she gave birth, as was feared, to a hydrocephalic baby.

The baby was seen by a paediatric surgeon who inserted a shunt in the area of blockage in the second week of life in order to relieve the blockage and so reduce the increased cerebrospinal pressure that had resulted. After extensive counselling both Shirley and her husband insisted that everything possible should be done for the baby. Shirley, although still very busy with her first baby, spent much time visiting her new baby and studying the disease, its complications and its possible outcome.

Shirley attended my rooms eight months later. None of the investigations and tests had indicated a specific cause for the baby's condition. We discussed future pregnancies and noted that Shirley had a 1 in 20 chance of another child having some form of neural tube defect (the neural tube is a tube formed of cells in very early life that will develop into the brain and spinal cord). Ultrasound had not at first revealed any abnormality and no reason could be given for the hydrocephaly.

We discussed the pregnancy, and I asked her if investigations, such as ultrasound and amniocentesis, had revealed an abnormality earlier in the pregnancy, would she have requested termination. "No", she replied, "I don't believe in terminations. I'm a Christian and believe abortion is murder." "What", I persisted, "if your life was at risk?" Shirley replied, "I would accept termination if both our lives were at risk. If one life can be saved then it's better to save one than to lose both." "What", I finally asked, "if the life of only one were at risk?" Shirley almost screamed, "No termination! Not even for a foetal abnormality!"

Shirley was a mother who had had many problems and suffered much hardship during the following eight months in dealing with and caring for the hydrocephalic baby who had undergone surgery. She had difficult nights and worked hard in caring for such a child. Coupled with this was the worry caused by the uncertainty of its future. Shirley also encountered a very negative attitude from members of society, such as the nurses, doctors, neighbours and friends, who discouraged her from persevering with treatment and operations. The most poignant occurrence was when her husband abandoned her. He found that his wife spent all her waking moments in worrying over and in caring for her baby. Family life as he understood it no longer existed. He could not tolerate it any longer.

Loving and caring for a severely handicapped baby, who was virtually condemned to death both prenatally and postnatally by much of society, had, remarkably, made Shirley appreciate her baby even the more.

How many "Shirleys" are there in our world who, despite their own beliefs and love, feel that they have to sacrifice their little ones because society refuses to accept these severely handicapped babies as an integral part of our society and our life?

It is appropriate here to say a little more about hydrocephaly. It is a condition where the head enlarges due to an abnormal collection of cerebrospinal fluid caused by an imbalance between its production and absorption. This leads to an enlargement of the ventricles in the brain which, in turn, exert pressure on the brain substance, and hence on the bones of the cranium. There are many types of hydrocephalus and many causes.

Congenital hydrocephaly is one of the most common abnormalities of the central nervous system and can occur alone, in association with spina bifida, or as part of a more complex disease, such as the Dandy-Walker Syndrome, which is a congenital malformation of the brain involving the cerebellum (an area at the back of the brain that controls movement) and the fluid filled spaces around it.

Shirley's baby suffered from the second variety, namely, hydrocephaly plus spina bifida (a congenital defect in the closure of the vertebral canal which allows the coverings of the spinal cord to protrude) Alpha feto-protein, which may be looked for in maternal serum early in the second trimester, is raised in all cases of congenital neurological disease, but is non-specific, and in any case, Shirley was not seen at that stage of pregnancy, and when ultrasound was carried out at the 22nd week, hydrocephaly was not noticed. In those days neurosurgical surgery was performed, appropriately, on Shirley's baby shortly after birth. Nowadays research is in progress to enable appropriate decompressive surgery to be undertaken in utero. This should improve prognosis enormously. It is being encouraged by those physicians who are actively interested in the welfare of the foetus in utero, and also by those parents who, because of their religion and their total rejection of late abortions, demand that something must be done to improve the chances of those neurologically damaged babies.

Hydrocephalus of non-infectious origin can obtain benefit from intraventricular decompression performed during the antenatal period. Much research is needed to improve diagnosis and treatment, and this is only possible if we consider the foetus to be a living, human being and, consequently, a patient. If diagnosis is made before the intracranial pressure causes brain damage then, theoretically at least, the outcome of decompression should be able to leave an unaffected baby, that is, one as healthy as a non-affected one.

Abortion as Contraception

I greeted Elizabeth in the waiting room of my Consulting Rooms, as was my usual custom, and gave her a smile. She had a bounce in her step when she stood up, but as she gazed at me a look of incredulity spread over her face and she appeared to wonder if she had, perhaps, made a mistake in coming to me for assistance. Was I going to help her?

She put on a stern expression and did not return my smile. After a few seconds she said, "I want an abortion." Looking over the questionnaire that she had filled in while waiting to see me I noticed that she worked in a Family Planning Centre. I began, therefore, by asking her if there had been some problem with her contraception. She answered with self-assurance and said that, in her teaching, abortion was one form of contraception. Continuing, she said, " I had a slight complication with the pill and therefore I chose the latter method." I tried to explain that termination of pregnancy also had its own complications.

She smiled in a way to suggest how ignorant I was and said, "Oh doctor, this is my fifth termination. On the contrary, in expert hands there is no risk. You see? I am the perfect example! We discussed all the options of family planning and this appeared to be the right thing for me. A woman has the right to do what she wants to with her own body."

I asked her if there were not moral and ethical risks in terminating a life. She said, "We advise people to terminate a pregnancy early when the foetus is not a human being. When it is merely a fertilized egg between a man and a woman." She appeared to be lecturing me with the hope, and even the expectation, of converting me to her point of view. She wanted me to carry out a procedure on her own terms and be convinced that what I was doing was right.

I always like to give the patient a chance to think deeply and to make a choice that is not harmful to herself or to others, so I said, "I should like to see you, with your husband, next week, and do an ultrasound to confirm the pregnancy and to confirm that it is also within the uterus and not an ectopic," She gasped and replied, "Doctor, by next week the foetus is that much bigger!" "So we have both come to the conclusion," I continued, "that the foetus growing inside you is alive, and has been from the moment of conception". She exhibited first astonishment and then dismay at my reasoning, but then said roughly, "The baby does not have human rights within the mother's womb". It was a terrible thought to realise that what she had just said was perfectly correct. The unborn baby has no rights under Law. As soon as it is born it is given rights, yet it is the same baby with the same DNA.

Since she was dealing with Family Planning and considered herself to be an expert in that regard, and since there was still a gulf between us, I attempted to span that chasm so that, if I could not dissuade her from having a termination, I could, at the least, convince her that her reasoning needed to be reviewed so that she could more honestly deal with the many women whom she counselled in the Family Planning Clinic. I told her that as it was her duty to advise the people whom she saw in the Family Planning Centre to the best of her ability, so it was my duty, under the law, to inform her of all the complications that could occur in those undergoing termination of pregnancy. This I did, and then asked her to print out the complications that I had enumerated and hand out copies to the people whom she saw in her clinic who might be considering abortion. I said, "You can only have a choice when you are well aware of all the implications".

Finally, I said, "As a Health Professional you should be educated and should educate and re-educate others". I told her, "I also am all for choice, but choice based on knowledge of all the facts. Those planning abortion should, first of all, consider all the facts. Research literature has convincingly shown that those choosing an abortion are more likely to have venereal disease, and, in particular be H.I.V. positive, than those having normal pregnancies. Obviously some things are outside the realm of choice, but no one would choose to have H.I.V.!" Towards the end of our conversation I thought Elizabeth became more thoughtful, and I hoped that, even if she herself went ahead with her expressed determination of having an abortion, then perhaps at least she might be more cautious in recommending it to others.

In my thirty-seven years of gynaecological practice I have seen many women who have requested abortion. I cannot give exact statistics, but I suggest that of those that I have counselled some 50% decided to maintain their pregnancies while the other 50% went elsewhere and had their pregnancies terminated. Many of the former patients subsequently declared that the baby they had contemplated destroying had become the most loved person in their lives. Of the latter, some 25% returned to me for treatment of complications resulting from the abortion that they had just had, or for future gynaecological consultations. It was interesting to note that they, apparently, had no desire to see again the doctor who had performed the abortion for them. Neither had they any wish to undergo further terminations.

Premature Baby

It was 7 o'clock on an autumn morning when I started my hospital rounds, which had to be finished before I saw my first patient at 9am in my Harley Street rooms. Beginning in the Maternity Ward I found, as usual, that Maria was not in her bed. She spent most of her time in the Intensive Care Baby Unit with her 28-week premature baby.

I found her with a blank expression on her face, gazing at her baby who was in an incubator with oxygen flowing in and with a naso-gastric feeding tube in place. The whole flow of Maria's life appeared to be frozen. Indeed, she had a vacant look and appeared to be quite unaware of her surroundings.

Maria was of Spanish descent. She was tall, with long, black hair tied at the back in an untidy fashion. I wanted to comfort her. The nursing staff told me that she was disconsolate and wept every night. I took Maria to her room and tried to hold a conversation with her.

She tried to rouse herself and started by saying that giving birth to a premature baby was quite different from having a full term baby. Her first pregnancy went like a breeze. The labour was easy and the baby was perfect. She continued, "Just as your body may go into physical shock after a serious accident, so having this premature birth, and seeing my baby connected up to all those tubes has given me an emotional shock. I feel numb and am

60

disconnected from what is going on around me. I feel my baby is in pain, and I don't understand what the doctors and nurses are telling me. I don't, in fact, believe what they are telling me."

Maria went into premature labour at the 28th week of gestation, in spite of medical treatment given to try to prevent such an eventuality. Her previous history was as follows: She had a full term pregnancy when she was 18-years-old. When her baby was only six months old she became pregnant again. She became distressed, cried for help and was advised to have a termination of the pregnancy. A surgical abortion was performed but she continued to bleed so a further evacuation of the uterus was carried out.

She planned to get pregnant again when her baby was two years old. Although she had no difficulty in getting pregnant, nevertheless, she could not maintain a pregnancy and had no less than three midtrimester spontaneous miscarriages. Investigations were undertaken and it was confirmed that she had an incompetent cervix, which is a weakened cervix that fails to retain the baby. It is a cause of miscarriage and preterm birth in the second and third trimesters. This had been explained to Maria, together with the conclusion that the cervix must have been damaged by the termination or the subsequent curettage.

Cervical circlage, the encirclement of the cervix by a stitch, is said to be successful in maintaining such a pregnancy in some 80 to 90% of such pregnancies but there is some risk of premature rupture of the membranes, infection and premature birth. The same complication, as has already been noted, occurred again in Maria's 5th pregnancy, even though cervical circlage was performed.

In spite of the tremendous advances that have occurred in the care and treatment of the premature baby there are still a number who suffer from serious medical conditions, or who will die, even though they may receive the best medical care available. Lasting disabilities, such as cerebral palsy, mental retardation and learning problems occur all too commonly in those born prematurely, even in those receiving the best medical care, although many do survive and grow up to be perfectly healthy.

I myself was always concerned with premature birth and I spent some time in Ruakura Animal Research Centre in New Zealand with Professor Sir Graham Liggins to undertake research into parturition (the process of childbirth) in cows and sheep. Although there has been immense progress, problems still arise and there is still no totally effective way to avoid prematurity.

Over the last two decades the incidence of prematurity has not decreased, rather it has increased. Prematurity is defined as birth before the 37th week of gestation. Obviously the older gestational age that the baby has, when born, the more favourable the outcome will be, especially with modern paediatric care. However, when the degree of prematurity nears 28 weeks or below then the future is precarious, and it follows that many such babies who survive will have life long disabilities requiring constant medical supervision and care. In the year 2001 7% of babies born in the U.K. were born prematurely. That means 45,000 babies were born prematurely out of 650,000 total births. In the U.S.A. one in eight babies are now born prematurely, that is more than 500,000 babies a year! According to one report from the U.S.A. premature birth has increased there by more than 30% over the last 20 years, and the cost of caring for those fragile infants has skyrocketed to 26 billion US dollars a year. The conclusion, of course, is that trauma occurring as a result of termination of pregnancy results in many more premature deliveries.

A final thought of Maria to whom I was speaking: Over the course of half an hour of intimate conversation she found that she could relax and tell me about all her fears. She recognized that the torn cervix had been responsible for all her misery. What had been responsible for the torn cervix? She at last understood. Had she not had that termination several years before then all her subsequent misery would have been spared. One hoped that having acknowledged the prime cause of her unfortunate predicament then, perhaps, she would be able to move forward.

Amniocentesis

Sarah, a Jewish lady from Israel, attended my consulting rooms requesting amniocentesis (aspiration of some of the fluid that the foetus lives in, by means of a needle inserted through the abdominal wall and uterus, with the object, usually,. to determine whether or not the foetus has a genetic disorder). She was 38 years old and pregnant for the first time. She was 12 weeks pregnant, and in view of her age, was obviously worried about her baby's health.

She was a very pleasant, broadminded, likeable person. She told me that she was a biblical scholar. This interested me, so I asked her what her reaction would be if some problem were discovered with the baby. She replied, "I would not want an abortion. I only want to be prepared in case something is amiss."

The fact that she volunteered that she was a biblical scholar made me curious to find out what the Torah said about induced abortion and what the general Jewish teaching was concerning such matters. She smiled and said that biblical teaching was clear but that its interpretation changed according to the fashion of the day. "Our way of life and fashions may change, but we are the same people as we were thousands of years ago. Biblical teaching makes sense. For instance, if I have an abortion because of some slight abnormality picked up by amniocentesis, I will be that much older when I next become pregnant, and then the risk will be even greater. Obviously, if amniocentesis showed that the baby had an abnormality incompatible with life then I might think further about it."

She then quoted passages of scripture to me that condemned termination of pregnancy. She said that the basic Jewish tenets concerned the sacredness of human life, the duty to populate the earth to ensure Jewish survival, and the Divine Presence, a deep sense of the sanctity of life in all it's manifestations and degrees, and a profound horror of blood and bloodshed. "These themes", she said, "underpin the entire Jewish approach to abortion". She continued, "The Jewish abhorrence of deliberate bloodshed and its respect for life, including that of the unborn, formed the natural foundation for the Christian view on abortion. The unborn child is a body and soul with a personal relationship with God".

"In that case", I replied, "there is always a slight risk that amniocentesis might cause a miscarriage. Perhaps it might be better if we performed a more simple, non-invasive test". This she gladly agreed to. She had an uneventful pregnancy and she gave birth to a full term, healthy baby with normal chromosomes.

It is noteworthy to record that she was upbraided by the midwife who was looking after her in her lying in period for daring to go through pregnancy without having had an amniocentesis. It is interesting to see how many modern day nurses and doctors follow the fashion, current at the time, without considering moral or personal reasons which might dictate an alternative point of view or treatment.

Breast Cancer and Termination of Pregnancy

Caroline had visited my Consulting Rooms on a number of occasions during the previous two or three years. A wealthy and popular figure, she said to me when she was 34 years old, "You know Doctor, I've not been taking the contraceptive pill for two years now and I still have not become pregnant. Do you think that there is anything wrong?"

I asked her if she wanted to get pregnant. "No, not at the moment", she replied, "although, at some time in the future I should like to have children". She had a very busy schedule and it was not then convenient. A full gynaecological examination failed to identify any abnormality so I reassured her. However I warned her that she was beginning to live, as far as conception was concerned, on borrowed time, that as soon as she could she should try to start a family, and that if pregnancy did not immediately follow I would then undertake some endoscopic exploratory investigations.

A year later she became pregnant and came requesting termination of the pregnancy. I explained that it was a most unwise thing to contemplate for someone who was thirty-five and also sub-fertile. Ultrasound confirmed that she was eight weeks pregnant. Although I attempted to dissuade her she was adamant and attended an abortion clinic where the termination was carried out.

One year later she developed breast cancer. She had surgery, radiotherapy and chemotherapy, with treatment extending over several months. Her greatest desire then was to complete her treatment and have a baby. Her oncologist, on the other hand, considered a breast cancer at that young age to be an extremely serious thing and that all one could hope for was the saving of the patient's life.

One only wished that one could have helped this patient. Did the early abortion enable the semi-matured breast cells, whose full maturation had been suspended by the early termination, to become more vulnerable to carcinogens than would have been the case if she had carried the foetus to term? We do not know.

Since breast cancer is the second most common cause of death in women today after cancer of the lung, it is necessary for me to say a little about this condition. It is well recognised that it is commoner in those who have not born children, and the fact that it was found to be more prevalent amongst nuns as far back as the 17th century would tend to confirm this. The first full-term pregnancy, especially if it occurs early in a woman's reproductive life, followed by breastfeeding, appears to offer some protection, while an early menarche (date of the first period) or late menopause (date of the last period) appears to increase the risk.

Besides endocrinological factors, genetic influences play a part, for it is well known that the condition runs in families. In addition, the disease occurs more commonly in the older age groups. Breast cells also are particularly sensitive to exposure to carcinogens. Finally, obesity may be an aetiological factor of which to take note, for a high intake of animal fat may, in some cases, especially in the elderly, also lead to the development of cancer of the breast.

The relationship between early abortion and breast cancer has been extensively studied since the 1950s and the answer is still uncertain. Earlier investigations suggested that there was a link between the two. However, more recent studies, based on medical histories taken from hospital records and not from self-reports, tended to refute this concept and several scientific bodies have generally adopted this latter view. Should this not be reassessed? Patients, as a rule, do not broadcast the fact that they have had abortions and often do not tell their parents, let alone their doctors; while abortion clinics are confidential, do not communicate with general practitioners, and do not follow up their patients. Hospital records alone, accordingly, are likely to give an entirely false result. It appears to me that the reasoning is flawed and more careful research is still required to find an answer to the question.

Breast Cancer and a Moral Dilemma.

Kathy was sitting on a chair opposite me with a smile of hope and trust lighting up her face. She started speaking, "I had major surgery recently for advanced breast cancer and am at present receiving chemotherapy. I should like to ask your advice about pregnancy. The doctor told me I should not get pregnant. He said that as a new pregnancy will make my condition deteriorate more rapidly, the pill is contra-indicated, and because the safe period is impossible, I am not to worry if I get pregnant but have an abortion."

In other words, the specialist had advised that the best form of contraception for her was termination of pregnancy should it inadvertently occur. This advice had caused her considerable distress and uncertainty and it was only her great faith in God which had enabled her to face each succeeding day, and care for her family.

In spite of treatment the cancer was spreading, and although her pale face and hollow cheeks lighted up from time to time as she thought of God she was sad and confused that the doctor should offer her treatment which was contrary to her belief.

I explained to her that although chemotherapy normally produced sterility and the cessation of the menses, or periods as people generally call them, yet it was still possible for an occasional ovulation to take place before completion of treatment.

She understood how dangerous would be the continuation of a pregnancy, not only for her but also for an unborn baby. However, she claimed that abortion under any circumstances is murder and no one should have the right to take another's life, particularly that of an innocent baby who is defenceless. That a mother and doctor, both of whom are expected to protect infant life, should collude to destroy it, seemed to her to be the height of immorality. "No," she concluded, "if you are to help me it must be before pregnancy has occurred."

It was decided, therefore, that surgical sterilisation on medical grounds be carried out, even though the risk of pregnancy occurring was remote.

It might be salutary to end this short report by saying a little about what is known of the effects of the female sex hormones on mammary cancers:

It has been known for many years that oophorectomy (removal of a patient's ovaries) will lead to regression of cancer of the breast. It has also more recently been shown that hormone replacement therapy (HRT) for the post-menopausal patient is more liable to be followed by the development of breast cancer than in those women who do not use HRT. For these reasons, and for others that take into account the time of the menarche (time of onset of the first period), the time of the first full term pregnancy and the onset of the menopause (time of cessation of the periods) all led scientists to presume that patients who developed breast cancer during pregnancy, or who became pregnant when suffering from cancer of the breast, had a much poorer prognosis. This, indeed, was the generally held view when this patient was seen.

Approximately 3% of breast cancers are associated with pregnancy or lactation, so the problem needs to be kept under review. The latest information available indicates that continuation of pregnancy does not appreciably affect the survival rate of such patients. In other words, the survival rate is the same as it is for pre-menopausal women with breast cancers of the same stage. In addition it has been shown that chemotherapy given to such women in the second half of pregnancy does not cause foetal abnormalities. Finally, the latest information comparing life expectancy of breast cancer patients having terminations with those who carry their pregnancies to term do not differ. In other words, termiation of pregnancy neither improves the outcome of patients with advanced cancer of the breast, nor does it make it worse.

It will be seen from this short case report that medical knowledge is developing and changing all the time, and doctors usually try their best to keep up with the latest knowledge, although in some cases they may be a few months late in acknowledging and accepting new ideas. It is perhaps also important that they listen to their patients, appreciate their fears and ethical beliefs, and try to tailor their proposed treatment to be acceptable, as far as is possble, to their patients' expectations.

'Our Little Miracle'

Clare was visibly shaking. Her head and eyes were lowered and she continued to lean on her husband's arm in spite of being seated opposite me. I looked at the referral letter. It read, "This 47-year-old postmenopausal woman has been vomiting for some time. She has lost weight and a tumour is growing within her abdomen". Clare's face was bloated and a look of despair spread over her countenance so that she looked much older than she actually was. Her eyes were reddened and her skin glistened with perspiration.

I glanced at her husband who was holding her hand. He too was sad and depressed. In fact, they were both without hope, and despair was expressed in their countenances.

I began by asking Clare to tell me her story. She sighed and said, "I am going through the change of life". She could go no further. Her voice croaked. She lowered her head and tried to collect herself. Still holding her husband's hand, she drew a deep breath and continued. "I started to feel sick and brought everything up. My doctor thought that HRT would help but it made me worse so I stopped it. I lost a lot of weight but, in spite of that, put on size in the middle so that now my tummy sticks out".

Questioning her further, I learnt that she had four grown up sons and that her husband had had a vasectomy ten years previously. She then said, "My youngest boy left home last year. We just led a quiet life and I had been planning to attend University" (This patient was seen in Sydney, Australia, where many middle-aged women entered Macquarie University as mature students after their children were grown up).

She continued, "For once I felt free from bringing up a family." Tears rolled down her cheeks. She sighed and said, "Now this has happened. It doesn't seem that I can make it now. I feel so weak and the lump in my tummy is growing so fast. I don't have any pain but I worry so much that I get a tightness in my chest". "What", I asked, "do you think it is?" She looked at me in amazement, as though pitying my stupidity, and replied, "Why what else can it be but cancer?"

In the three or four minutes that Clare had been in my office she had worked herself up into a state of great frenzy. I tried to calm her down by asking her to lie on the examination couch and take deep breaths. She gradually relaxed and her breathing slowed. I then examined her abdomen. This revealed a uterus enlarged to the size of a 22 week gestation. I had an ultrasound in my consulting room. This I applied, and it confirmed an active 22-week-foetus with a strong heart beat. I called her husband in and the three of us gazed at the sight with amazement. They both gasped in surprise, and a feeling of relief was obvious. Clare burst out laughing and expressed her delight that it was not cancer.

Obviously their immediate surprise and joy might be short lived when they came to think about the future and all the questions that would arise, so I sent them home with the instruction that they should become accustomed to the new situation and return to see me in a week's time when I should be happy to answer all their questions. I also gave them a pamphlet that I had written for my elderly pregnant patients about their specific situation.

Clare duly returned in a week's time. She came alone, and on this occasion she was upright, had a smile on her face, and appeared to be like a conqueror. She began by saying, "I had the most unusual week of my life; not only me but the whole family. We had discussion after discussion. I thought that I was condemned to death by a growing cancer. I had thought that my hopes of seeing my grandchildren were over; as was my ambition to study Art at University. I married young. I never went to University for I had a family to look after. I always loved Art. I was looking forward to the time when I should be free". Words tumbled out of her mouth as she tried to express her emotions.

She continued, "First we opened a bottle of Champaign to celebrate that I didn't have cancer. But I still had a lump in my tummy. I was shocked that at my age I was having a baby. I read the brochure that you gave me. How could I face friends and family? How could I face society as a whole? Sometimes I thought that I had escaped execution only to fall a victim to slavery. I would be stuck at home for the rest of my life".

"This lump must still be malignant, whatever way I looked at it", she reasoned, "I thought the simplest way would be to get rid of it so I rang an abortion clinic and made an appointment to see them. They were so sympathetic and confirmed my thinking that it was out of the question for me to have a baby at my age. The only problem is that it will be a lot of money to pay. In the meantime, since I had arranged to see you, I thought you might be able to help me to get it paid for by the insurance".

She continued, "Something else also happened. I felt the baby move. I thought about the days when I had had my children. During the last week I haven't slept properly as all these thoughts are going round and round in my head. I wish someone else would make the decisions for me. Can't you help me?"Clare asked me to go through the pamphlet that I had given her which discussed the various problems that could arise for those of advancing age who become pregnant. She had, of course, already read it but had become even more confused; so we read it together:

We read about the increased risk of having a genetic disorder, such as Down's Syndrome, which causes mental retardation, and defects of the heart and other organs due to the presence of an additional chromosome.

Secondly, we discussed the increased risk of miscarriage, often precipitated by the presence of a genetic abnormality.

Next we discussed various medical conditions such as pre-eclampsia (a disease of pregnancy associated with high blood pressure, swelling of the legs and often other parts of the body as well, and protein in the urine), high blood pressure, diabetes, accidental haemorrhage (intrauterine bleeding other than that caused by premature placental separation that may occur when the placenta is low lying) and intrauterine growth retardation (inadequate foetal growth), all of which are commoner in the more elderly patient.

Finally we discussed labour with the complications that are more likely to occur, such as prolonged labour, the greater need for Caesarean section, and the greater risk of postpartum haemorrhage (bleeding from the uterus after the child has been born).

It became apparent that Clare was not now worried about herself, for she had overcome cancer and death. What she really wanted to know was if the baby was normal. She was still undecided what to do.

I carried out a more detailed ultrasound scan and was glad to see that there were no obvious abnormalities. She was much more relaxed and even smiled when she saw her baby sucking her thumb. Indeed, she was really quite delighted when she realized that she was carrying a baby girl. She said, "I have four sons and I always wanted to have a daughter". Her main desire by now was for reassurance. I said to her that in modern times, now that more women were playing more important roles in the market place, they were putting off having their families until later, so that now it was quite common for women not to have their babies until after the age of thirty. I further added that although her advanced age, as far as childbirth was concerned, was a disadvantage medical science has also advanced since she had had her family so that perhaps the risk of a mishap was not as great as she feared. I suggested that if I carried out amniocentesis for her it would be possible to be able to exclude the one really serious condition that she could encounter, namely Down's Syndrome.

All this was too much for Clare to digest. Having got rid of a growing cancer which threatened her life, she was now faced with a growing baby. She said, "It's all like a nightmare. I'm still in a hazy dream". I said, "Although there are many things that could complicate your pregnancy medical science has moved forward and we are that much better at being able to detect and deal with them when they arise". By this time I thought I ought to involve the husband so I made a further appointment to see the couple together.

It so happened that the following week coincided with her 47th birthday. Apparently her husband had arranged a surprise party for a 'dying wife'. Her four sons were there to comfort their mother, and then the husband made the surprised announcement that his wife was expecting their fifth child and there was general rejoicing. The sons all insisted that their little sister should be called Sheila, so that was the toast.

All this made my discussion with the pair much easier. Clare said that the decision not to have an abortion was not difficult. "I just couldn't have lived with the fact that I could, so easily, have destroyed a life", she declared. "It would have been a decision that my husband and I would have bitterly regretted to the end of our days".

I asked them if they wanted to go ahead and have the amniocentesis performed. Clare replied, "As we're not going to have an abortion, and since there's no medical treatment for Down's Syndrome anyway, what would be the point in you doing an amniocentesis?" Her reasoning was perfect, so we simply decided closely to monitor the pregnancy and to keep a careful watch for any signs of growth retardation.

At term we decided to deliver the baby by Caesarean Section and carry out tubal ligation at the same time, on her request. We invited the husband to be present at the delivery. He was so delighted and said, "I was never allowed to be present at the births of my other children. This is something that I shall treasure all my days".

The day for the elective Caesarean section was arranged, as was the decision that it should be performed under epidural anaesthesia (a kind of spinal anaesthetic in which the patient is awake). On that momentous occasion the operation was performed with the husband sitting near his wife's head and holding her hand. It truly was a joy for all to behold when a healthy little girl was delivered and shown to Clare.

At the sixth week postnatal visit Clare said, "We have an adorable little girl whom we all love dearly. The boys all think she's great. She has given us all something to think about and has brought out the best in all of us. We've become a more closely knit family and are looking forward to the challenge of seeing her grow up".

Clare saw me a year later. I asked about Sheila. She said, "We all love her very much and just couldn't imagine life without her". She had also managed to arrange to study Art at Macquarie University. The baby was her model and she was continually drawing her in different positions!

Psychiatric Disorder; a Medical Misdiagnosis

T he reason for including this case is not that she had an abortion, but that she might well have had a termination to save her life because it was thought that she had a disease of pregnancy that threatened her very existance. However the true medical condition was eventually recognized.and so termination was averted.

Frances was admitted via the Casualty Department with severe vomiting. She was 21 years of age, came from Eastern Europe, and was not an easy patient to understand or to deal with. She was withdrawn, pale and dehydrated. Her mouth was so dry that she could barely speak. There was also considerable difficulty in understanding her for she spoke little English, and her story was eventually taken with the aid of an interpreter. There was no history of a vomiting or eating disorder. She was about two months pregnant and ultrasound confirmed a singleton pregnancy (a single foetus—severe vomiting in pregnancy is much commoner in cases of multiple pregnancy). Although she had not planned the pregnancy, nevertheless, she was quite happy with the knowledge. Examination revealed her to be undernourished and extremely ketotic (a condition in which an abnormal increase of ketones in the blood occurs and which if not adequately treated can be life-threatening). When the blood sugar drops, and the body does not have suffecient stored carbohydrates to correct the problem, it converts fats into usable carbohydrates, a process called gluconeogenesis, to meet energy needs. Ketones are byproducts of this process.

We know that nausea affects between 70 and 85% of women in early pregnancy and that actual vomiting occurs in 50%. Indeed, it is almost considered to be of normal occurrence. Beginning usually about the ninth week of gestation it has usually settled by the twelfth week. In some cases, however, it is so persistent and severe that it causes weight loss, dehydration and ketosis. To this is given the name of hyperemesis gravidarum.

Frances was admitted to the ward and given fluid, dextrose and electrolytes by intravenous drip, as well as anti-emetics (drugs used to treat vomiting). Although her general condition improved, vomiting recurred whenever she was discharged from hospital and continued well after the twelfth week of pregnancy. Indeed, her condition was such that fear was expressed for her life and it was suggested to her that it might be necessary to terminate the pregnancy to avoid such a catastrophe, but this she declined.

During my daily hospital visits Frances never returned my smile and she continued to be withdrawn. This was attributed to the language problem. The hospital staff and I were, nevertheless, still very concerned about the lack of communication until, one day, one of the nurses caught her self-inducing the vomiting. A psychiatric opinion was therefore urgently sought.

The psychiatrist confirmed that Frances was suffering from anxiety and depression so he prescribed suitable medication. Her vomiting slowly decreased and finally ceased altogether, and her mood improved. She was eventually discharged, needed no further hospital admissions until she went into labour at the 37th week and gave birth to a healthy, male infant whom the paediatrician confirmed as being entirely normal. The psychiatrist continued to see her during her lying in period and beyond, for he feared that she might develop postnatal depression, but nothing sinister occurred.

This was an unusual case in that, due to lack of communication, a psychiatric disorder was at first missed. The initial diagnosis of severe hyperemesis gravidarum, not responding to treatment, and where termination of the pregnancy might be required to save the woman's life, was much commoner in the days when Frances was seen than it is today, possibly because nowadays intravenous and electrolyte therapy are more rigorously monitored and enforced. Nevertheless, in exceptional cases it might still need to be considered. The disease is normally confined to the first trimester, and although it appears to be associated with rising hormone levels the exact pathogenesis (the origin and course of development of disease) has still not been discovered. Further research is required to fully elucidate the problem.

Secondly, it needs to be stressed that psychiatric disorders are more common in pregnancy than are generally recognised. The psychiatrist claimed that about 20% of pregnant women suffer from either minor, or sometimes major, depressive, or bipolar disorders which, if not treated, pose substantial risks to the mother and child. He continued, "Pregnant women can suffer from the same illnesses as those who are not pregnant, and, in spite of the longstanding notion that pregnancy is a time of happiness and emotional well-being, some suffer from depression and anxiety." Finally he said that in the past doctors used to be very wary of prescribing psychiatric medication to pregnant women, but that nowadays more information is available about the effect of various psychiatric drugs on the foetus and, consequently, more pregnant women are able to continue with their treatment.

Asherman's Syndrome

Susan was an attractive twenty-three-year-old American who worked in an oil company. Sitting opposite me with her lovely brown eyes looking at the floor, her long hair covering her shoulders, and her hands clasped together she said, "Doctor, I've not been able to conceive. I've been trying for two years but nothing has happened." She heaved a big sigh. "I had no difficulty in getting pregnant when we first got married, but we were in the process of building up a home and it was just not convenient. I didn't know it would happen to me. I had a short consultation and counselling, and, before I could think about it, I found myself in the operating theatre. I had a sense of relief when I awoke after the termination and I thought I should be able to start a new life. But I continued to bleed for three weeks and had to have a D and C (Dilatation and Curettage). It was only when I found that I couldn't conceive that I had doubts about the abortion and started to read books about it."

Susan was an intelligent young lady who not only read books to try to solve her problem, but also made extensive use of the internet. This is an extremely good way to investigate a problem, provided one realises that when researching a controversial subject the information one obtains will be biased by the scientist's point of view.

Continuing she said, "I know that in our Western culture the sanctity of human life is enshrined in our laws, but early pregnancy cannot be human life, and that, I suppose, is why abortion is legal. I was only eleven weeks pregnant. I discovered that 1.29 million abortions took place in the U.S.A. in 2002, so it must have been O.K. for a further one to have been added. Surely it can't be wrong if every one's doing it? I'm puzzled why there are different laws in the different States in America when it becomes illegal for abortions to be carried out, for surely that should be when the pregnancy becomes human, but the thought is deep in my mind. From time to time, when I think about it, I feel guilty and have a sense of loss, but I tell myself that it was only blood clot and a piece of jelly and that I can start again. Unfortunately, however, I've been trying for the last two years without success, and thoughts about the abortion keep nagging me. Doctor, I really want a baby!"

A thorough investigation of Susan revealed that she had Asherman's Syndrome, a condition in which curettage has removed some or all of the lining of the womb, thus allowing its inner surfaces to stick together.

For those unfamiliar with Asherman's Syndrome it might be worthwhile saying a little more about it. It is best described as a syndrome in which intrauterine adhesions or synechiae have formed as a result, usually of trauma, although rarely infection may be implicated. This can cause amenorrhea (cessation of periods) or hypomenorrhea (scanty periods), habitual abortion, and secondary infertility.

Most commonly intrauterine adhesions occur after dilatation and curettage performed because of a miscarriage or a placenta retained, with or without hemorrhage, after a delivery. Should the patient continue to bleed after such an occurrence and curettage becomes necessary, the basal lining of the interior of the uterus is particularly liable to be damaged, which results in the front and back surfaces of the uterus sticking together and becoming adherent. Occasionally the whole cavity of the uterus is obliterated, but more commonly, adhesions only form in a part, or parts, of the uterus. Adhesions sometimes also occur due to other conditions, such as after an elective abortion, after Caesarean section, and after uterine surgery, such as the removal of fibroids (benign uterine tumours). The extent of the adhesions defines whether the case is considered to be mild, moderate, or severe.

Asherman's Syndrome is thought to be under-diagnosed because it is usually undetectable by straightforward diagnostic procedures such as ultrasound scan. Hysterography was the older method of diagnosis, but hysteroscopy is more commonly employed nowadays and is more reliable.

Modern treatment is performed by an experienced hysteroscopist and laser surgeon who divides the adhesions. In all but the milder cases it is wise for the uterus also to be viewed during the procedure through the laparoscope to make sure that the intra-uterine surgery has not damaged any extra-uterine organs. Sequential oestrogen-progestogen therapy is often subsequently given to encourage regrowth of the endometrium (oestrogen and progesterone are hormones produced by the ovary that develop the lining of the uterus each month).

When I started medicine forty years ago, I was told that Asherman's Syndrome was very rare or non-existent. The first case that for me proved unequivocally that there was such a condition, was when I viewed an opened uterine specimen after hysterectomy. This finding became common after I had access to the hysteroscope. It is now recognised that Asherman's Syndrome is of worldwide distribution, and it has become more common since abortion has been liberalised.

It is interesting to note, in Susan's case, that the subsequent curettage, required because of continuing bleeding following her termination and subsequent very scanty periods, did not alert her medical attendant to the possibility that she might have Asherman's Syndrome. Due to the fact that an ordinary gynaecological examination will not reveal the condition, Susan lost three years of her fertility opportunity.

I carried out hysteroscopy and separation of the adhesions for her by laser and inserted an intrauterine contraceptive device at the end of the operation to keep the internal surfaces apart while healing was occurring. I also thought it wise to give her sequential oestrogen-progesterone to further encourage the reparative process. Susans's periods reverted to normal, but it took another two years before she became pregnant. She was warned that the pregnancy would need to be carefully monitored to make sure that any difficulties that arose could be expeditiously dealt with, since it is known that those who have had Asherman's Syndrome are more likely to face a variety of complications.

A Question of Guilt

arol, aged 36, was referred to me because she had not had any periods for three years. Two years previously she had had some investigations and had been told that she had reached the menopause.

She dated her complaint to an accident which had occurred three years previously when she had fallen over and had fractured her coccyx (the lowest bones in the spine). She suffered from severe anxiety, agoraphobia and had failed to obtain any happiness in the marriage situation.

Carol began by talking about her guilty feelings. She could not forgive herself. Eight years before she had been found to have a non-functioning right kidney. This was removed and the surgeon suggested that to prevent putting undue strain on the remaining kidney she should not get pregnant; therefore she had had her uterine tubes ligated. This upset her considerably.

I asked, "What do you feel guilty about?" Gazing at the floor she replied, "A year after the tubal ligation I thought I had become pregnant. I spoke to the gynaecologist who had done the sterilization but he just laughed at me, and it was only when I was having a follow up X-ray of my remaining kidney that it was confirmed that I really was pregnant. I went back to the gynaecologist and he advised me to have a termination straight away".

As Carol was telling her story her voice became louder and

self-accusatory. Continuing she said, "I never wanted to face reality". She had played a lot of fantasy games with herself and never allowed herself to believe that it really was a baby. "I knew, of course, that it was. I felt the life inside me. Every pregnant woman knows it. I wanted somebody to tell me it was just a bit of blood clot and jelly. Yes, that's what it was: blood clots and jelly. I convinced myself, so I happily went ahead. People use jelly for desert, but it never talks or walks."

Then Carol told me that she had a deep belief in reincarnation. She smiled and said, "My baby will have another chance". Then she frowned and said, "I can't forget what I've done".

I collected my thoughts and tried to decide how I could help her, for she was destroying herself. Carol herself sat motionless. "Can you go back over the events and tell me exactly what happened?" I asked. She did not appear to remember much of the detail but, all the time, she indulged in self-torture with her feelings of guilt. I gathered that she had had an unstable childhood and had hoped to have a loving family to compensate for that. Her husband had not been sympathetic. He had not shared her dilemma. He had merely said that it was her body and it was entirely her decision what she did. He had no concept or apparent concern for her subsequent guilty feelings. Carol said, "What is wrong with the world? Is there not one person in the world who understands me? Everyone just says you should forget it". It was obvious that Carol was plagued by feelings of guilt and mistrust, and a fear of others; for as Shakespeare has written:

> Suspicion always haunts the guilty mind;
> the thief doth fear each bush and officer.

Carol expressed deep rage which she directed at her husband. I could only sit and listen, and, from time to time, attempt to reassure her that she was expressing very human feelings.

I posed the questions: "Has your husband always been difficult? What happens, in other respects, in your married life?" She thought carefully about what I had asked and then said, "It's quite good in everything else. It's just for the abortion that he has no time. He doesn't carry the guilt that I do." She continued, "It was my choice and he left all the decisions to me. How can I carry such a load of guilt all my life alone?"

As was often the case in such psychologically difficult cases, I attempted to get her to agree to see a counsellor. I also tried to remind her of the alleged reason for which she had been referred i.e. the absence of periods. She confessed that her great wish was to have the tubal ligation reversed and have a baby.

I am glad to say that after some psychotherapy and further hormonal investigation it transpired that shock had been responsible for her amenorrhoea (absent periods) and her periods resumed. We discussed the trauma to which she had been subjected, and she it was who suggested to me that her ordeal should be published to act as a warning to others to help them to avoid such a catastrophe.

Feelings of Guilt

Jane, a 20-years-old Australian, engaged to be married, had last attended my consulting rooms two years previously. Originally she had seen me for a gynaecological problem, but after that she had become pregnant and I had delivered her of a little girl.

When she entered the room I had difficulty in recognising her at first, although I had delivered her of a baby two years previously. Her eyes were puffy and red, and she gazed at the floor whilst speaking. She suddenly burst into tears and said that she had had a termination three weeks previously.

She presented me with a screwed up piece of paper from an abortion clinic. This was a printed paper, presumably printed in thousands, with a name, and a circle around "general anaesthetic" and "ten-week-size pregnancy". I looked at Jane and asked her, "What is the problem?" She was silent and very pale, and a tear rolled down her cheek. After a further silence she said, "It didn't worry me at first, but as time passed......" She sighed and tears poured down her cheeks.

I was rather embarrassed as I did not know my real role here. Was I acting as a mother, dear friend, psychiatrist or gynaecologist? To relieve the situation, I looked around the room for some tissues as, by this time, Jane had completely dissolved in tears. I asked her what exactly happened. "I had a row with my financé," she replied. "He wanted to live in South Australia and I wanted to stay in Sydney with my parents, so I left him. I couldn't go through with it, and I didn't tell Mum. I rang the Family Planning Clinic and they put me in touch with the abortion centre. This happened so quickly. I went there. I had the termination and three hours later I went home." "Did you have any counselling?" I asked her. "Yes", she replied. "They told me that it was my body and that every woman should be able to do as she liked with her own body. I was told that one of the complications was infection, and that it would be prevented by a course of antibiotics." At that time Jane seemed quite able to accept the philosophy that a woman has the right to do as she wishes with her own body.

To my question, "How do you feel?" she replied, "It didn't affect me in the beginning but now," (and she started to cry again), "as time passes I feel I killed my baby." "Do you have pain? Are you still bleeding?" I asked. "Yes" she replied. However, Jane did not appear to be at all concerned about herself, her only concern and thought was for the baby.

Jane then said, "I keep telling myself: I had the right to do what I wanted with my own body. Then I thought: when one is angry one could do anything with one's body, but if I attempted to commit suicide everyone would stop me. I was angry with my fiancé. I wanted help. I wanted a sympathetic ear. I was desperate. I wanted to cut my wrists. If I went to the doctor and asked him to help me to cut them, would he have helped me? No! That would have been against the law. Why did he not stop me having an abortion? I can't understand the rationality that I can do what I want with my body. Why was there such a rush?"

Certainly Jane was not the same bubbly girl that I had known. Was she upset because of her financé, or was she suffering from post-abortal depression, or were there feelings of guilt, or a combination of all three? Certainly Jane needed to talk to someone and pour out her thoughts.

I was quite concerned about Jane for she felt very guilty about her action, and the feeling of guilt is a powerful one. She felt responsible, she felt condemned, she felt that she deserved punishment. She was depressed and unable to relate to people. I naturally thought that it really needed to be sorted out, so I continued by asking Jane whether she had ever suffered from depression in the past? She remembered that when she was 16 years old her parents had separated; she became very depressed and was given medication for three months. I therefore became even more concerned for two reasons: Firstly, I remembered reading about a Seventeenth-century British Bishop, Robert South, who wrote, "Guilt upon the conscience, like rust upon iron, both defiles and consumes it, gnawing and creeping into it, as that does which at last eats out the very heart and substance of the metal." Secondly, it is known that termination of pregnancy can cause post-abortal depression in people with a history of depression in the past. In Jane's case I had no hesitation, in requesting the assistance of a psychiatrist.

In attempting to understand post-abortal depression I first of all consulted the published literature on the subject. It has generated considerable media interest and medical research in recent years but unfortunately the results and conclusions reached differ wildly.

I therefore approached the Pregnancy Advisory Service that provides abortion services for women in Britain to enquire about the incidence of post-abortal depression amongst their clients, and was told that from their observation termination of pregnancy does not cause subsequent depression, provided the woman has discussed her options and has made an informed choice. Their spokeswoman went on to say, "Very few women return for post-abortion counselling because most have made the best decision for themselves at the time and see no further need to talk to a counsellor." Questioning her further about their 'follow up' procedure, I was told, "We do not follow up our patients. They are given a note to take to their doctor." Finally, I asked her what proportion of patients were referred by their General Practitioners.

She replied, "We really do not keep statistics, but most of our patients are self-referred." I thus concluded that I was not going to obtain any worthwhile statistical information from that quarter.

Speaking next to a Pro-Life Organization I was told that most of their patients who requested abortion either had financial hardship or had abusive male partners or were unmarried. The speaker went on to say that if the woman then decided to solve her immediate problem by having an abortion that also became a further source of trauma. Consequently, she feared that nearly all patients who had had terminations of pregnancy suffered from post-abortal depression.

It appeared that pro-choice supporters believed that post-abortal depression rarely, if ever, occured, while those who opposed termination of pregnancy believed that few, if any, who had had induced abortions escaped. I decided, therefore, to discuss the matter with a counsellor and psychiatric colleague of mine. He gave as his opinion that post-abortal trauma had traditionally been regarded as a specific form of post-traumatic stress disorder. The woman experiences the abortion event. There is then a latency period during which she appears to cope well. This is then followed by a cluster of symptoms which include intrusive trauma, a persistent sense of numbness, sleep disturbance, anxiety, depression, and suicidal feelings. Unfortunately, at this period of time, the patient may have actually forgotten about the abortion, or, due to a psychological, self-protective mechanism, that includes denial, and the unwillingness to recall the unpleasant experience, she may not recognize the symptoms for what they are. "For these reasons," he said, "it is not surprising that it is so difficult to get reliable information about post-abortal depression."

Data collected from my own patients' medical files indicate that, for many, a termination of pregnancy is nothing more than an act of despair. For all, it is an intense, emotional issue that irreversably changes the course of their lives and which reaches to the very depths of their sexuality and self-image. It must be remembered, too, that many women also suffer from depression after spontaneous abortion, and even after child bearing; but my own records also reveal that depression is much higher after termination, and may even occur ten years later. Indeed, in one case it was found to have occurred seventeen years later.

Burning Tummy Syndrome

Francis, a 41-year-old English woman living in Australia, hesitatingly looked round as she entered the room and shut the door. She sat down and said, "It's no better; I can't quite understand it. It's still burning." Francis presumed that I already knew her entire history and all about her problems. I must say that this was the first communication I had had with her. Neither had I been given a letter or any information about her.

I was rather taciturn on account of my ignorance, so I asked, "How long have you had problems?" "Only since the termination," she replied.

By this time Francis's mouth was quite dry and she rubbed her hands together. Sitting very tensely she became anxious and her hands shook slightly. She attempted to swallow and said, "Doctor, it's terrible. My mouth is so dry I can hardly speak." Not wishing to interrupt Francis I rang for a glass of water for her. She continued, "I wasn't well; I had a small marital problem so I went to the doctor and he suggested a termination. I felt terrible, but immediately went and had it done. I had no time to think or, rather, at that moment I couldn't think. I felt terrible. The burning sensation started and the pain was added to that of my varicose veins. I didn't want to get pregnant again so the doctor tied my tubes. I went back to him complaining of bleeding, pain and burning, and I was terrible; exactly as I am now. My problems increased and I went back two weeks later. I was crying with the pain and this burning feeling, so a hysterectomy was carried out. That was six weeks ago. The burning is all over my tummy and in the front and back passage. Really, doctor, it's all over ....." Francis's mouth was, by this time, quite parched, and the shaking of her hands had increased. She did not know how to sit comfortably and all the time she looked round to see if anybody else could hear her story.

I thought that if Francis lay on the examination couch it would enable her to relax and she might then be able to give me a better description of her symptoms. This she did, but she continued to complain of burning all over. I asked her to map out the area and she frowned, as if to say, "I am burning as though I were in a burning fire. How is it that you can't even see it or feel it?" She reluctantly put her hand all over her abdomen and pointed to her vagina, rectum and umbilicus.

When I examined her, I found a small umbilical hernia, a tender granulation in the vaginal vault and a haemorrhoid. As a matter of fact, however, she was not relaxed and therefore her whole abdomen appeared to be tender.

It was obvious that Francis was suffering from a state of anxiety, so it was all the more necessary to exclude concurrent physical disease. I told her that I would be in touch with her doctor and I made an appointment to see her again with her husband. At this stage Francis burst into tears and said, "Doctor, you must help me. I can't sleep or eat. I can't cope with my every day life and my marriage is hanging by a thin thread."

I decided to admit Francis to hospital and I arranged a combined specialist consultation. I called a surgeon and a psychiatrist, and I interviewed her husband. I visited Francis in hospital every day and she was gradually able to tell me her entire story. How dreadfully guilty she felt! By having operation after operation she thought she could sweep the trouble away.

After her uterus had been removed her gastro-intestinal tract occupied her thoughts. A Barium enema and endoscopy did not, however, reveal any abnormality and laparoscopy was also negative.

Francis's symptoms unfortunately continued. The psychiatrist visited her daily and treated her with anti-depressants. During treatment she was sleepy and calmer.

Whilst a patient in hospital Francis talked about her abortion and the effect it had had on her life, and on the relationship with her husband, her children, the neighbours, and the church. She thought that all the world knew about it and condemned her. She continued, "I wish it had never happened. I wish I had been given some time to think, or at least, I wish I had been counselled. I am guilty, of course. Because I had grown up children and very bad varicose veins the doctor advised that I should not get pregnant again. That was ten years ago. We had just started to build a home and we were working hard to get it finished. When I found myself pregnant I was shocked and rushed to the doctor, saying 'I can't cope.' By the next day everything was all over and finished. In that state I needed help and guidance. If the doctor had told me to throw myself off the Harbour Bridge I would have done it. I wanted support at that time. Now I have my home finished but I can't enjoy it. I'm burning day and night. I think it must be my bowel as my womb is out."

Extensive medical investigations failed to reveal a physical cause for her symptoms, and certain other symptoms were also uncovered during the course of the search, such as shortness of breath, palpitations and imsomnia. She required long term counselling, and was reported, towards the end of one of those sessions, to have remarked that it was a pity that she had not received such help before she had embarked upon that ill-fated termination.

Perforation of the Uterus

Early one morning I was battling through dense traffic to reach the hospital, where I had a full list of patients to see, when my bleep sounded. Normally I would have pulled over to the side of the road to speak to the hospital on my mobile phone but on that particular day the number of vehicles was such that it was impossible. I therefore spoke to the hospital while driving and learnt to my dismay that a young woman had been admitted to the hospital in a state of shock, was bleeding heavily, and would I see her immediately on my arrival.

I had scarcely finished receiving the message when the telltale noise of a police car siren sounded. The car ranged up alongside and I was ordered to pull over. Already disturbed by the message that I had just received, this unwelcome attention of the police was the last straw. They, of course, were doing their job, but so was I. Previously the British Medical Association had issued badges to members, and the police had allowed them leeway, but these had now been withdrawn. Was I to be fined for this misdemeanour? I breathlessly explained the state of affairs to the police. They fortunately believed me and wave me on, but I had wasted several minutes of valuable time.

On arriving in the hospital I was led to a small curtained-off area in the Outpatients' Department. There on a bed lay a young woman of nineteen years. She lay silently with her eyes closed and with her face as white as the pillow under her head. I spoke softly to her. She slowly opened her wonderful eyes, and, looking at me with a sense of desperation and lonely suffering, told me that she had been travelling, had become pregnant, and had had a termination in an Abortion Clinic in Paris. She had pain and continued to bleed but had been told that that was to be expected for a few days. It was only when her symptoms did not clear up and she appeared to be getting weaker by the day that, in desperation, she flew back to London, went to stay with a friend who brought her to the private hospital where I was working that day. This girl obviously was seriously ill so I asked who her next of kin was. She replied that it was her father, her mother having recently died, but she said that on no account was he to be told the nature of her illness.

She had a high temperature and a brief examination revealed that she was still bleeding vaginally, while abdominal examination indicated that she had peritonitis and was almost certainly bleeding internally as well. Blood was take for haemoglobin estimation, white cell count and group and cross-match, for she urgently needed a blood transfusion. Her haemoglobin level was found to be only 6gm/dl while the white blood count confirmed that she had a polymorpho-leucocytosis (high white cell blood count indicative of infection).

I never felt the responsibility of my profession more than I did that day. I had a full clinic for the morning and an operating list in the afternoon so it would be difficult to fit in a complicated case as well. Nevertheless, it was essential that she be taken to theatre as soon as the cross-match had been completed, blood was up and running into a vein, and an intravenous antibiotic was being administered. Clinic patients were cancelled, a surgical colleague kindly made his theatre available and an anaesthetist was summonsed.

Emergency laparotomy revealed two large perforations in the uterus and the pelvic cavity was found to be filled with blood and clot. This was evacuated, the rents in the uterus repaired, and then careful examination of the bowel undertaken to exclude damage. Having assured myself that the bleeding had been controlled and that there was no damage to bowel or other pelvic organs I breathed more freely for it is well known that undetected bowel damage is often the cause of death of such patients.

The preliminary resuscitation and operation had delayed everyone for about two hours, much to the annoyance, I am sure, of some of the patients and doctors. Most however were very understanding when it was explained to them that the operation was urgently needed to save life.

Sarah, the young lady about whom I have been writing, had a fairly stormy convalescence but was eventually discharged fit and well. Her father, a very honourable, though strict, elderly gentleman in his late sixties was very concerned for Sarah and tried to find out the cause of his daughter's illness. I had to explain to him that doctors were only trusted by their patients because, like priests in a confessional, they never divulged their patients' confidences or diseases without permission. He was not very happy with my reasoning, but to pacify him I said that I was sure that, when Sarah was better, she would talk to him herself, and with that he had to be content.

At the six weeks follow up examination Sarah told me the whole story. It seemed that she had for so long refrained from confiding in any living creature that she just had to speak to someone as a form of catharsis. I already knew more about her problems than anyone else but otherwise had no connection with her at all. This probably explains why she never came to see me again. She had made her confession and wished to move on.

After assuring me that she was feeling much better she began to unburden herself of her guilty feelings. This was obviously going to take some time and I was a little anxious that it would involve keeping other patients waiting. Nevertheless, I decided that it would be wrong to cut short her story if she were to obtain benefit from its disclosure. Continuing she said, "My mother and I were very close. Indeed, I was never afraid to tell her any of my

97

problems. She was like a sister to me and I had complete faith in her judgement and in any advice that she gave. She always stood by me, even when I made a mess of things as so many teenagers do. Sadly however she had been battling against breast cancer for a number of years and she finally passed away last year, just after I had finished my A Levels."

"What about your father?" I queried, "He has been terribly concerned about you and was a constant visitor when you were sick in hospital. "My father," she replied, "although kind and considerate is very restrictive and old fashioned, and I was never able to have any meaningful fellowship with him. However, when mummy died he did appreciate how devastated I was and, hoping to cure my depression, arranged for me to spend some time on a cruise ship during my gap year before I entered University to study Engineering and Design."

She fell silent as she remembered the event, and then continued, "The first night at sea I had the boat deck to myself although there were ninety first class cabin passengers. I was thinking about my mother and how I had often done things that had upset her, yet now I would have laid down my life for her. I remembered how she stood by me and loved me in spit of the many things I did to hurt her. I was so full of misery that I scarcely noticed that a storm had arisen. The ship started to pitch and toss and then the rain bucketed down so I went below and turned in. I couldn't sleep. The ship rocked and groaned and I lay in my bunk and recalled all the unhappy nights of past years. The storm without was nothing as compared with the storm within my own soul."

She paused to collect herself and then continued, "The storm had abated somewhat by the following morning so I went on deck where I got talking to a middle-aged man whose wife had divorced him. He was sad and lonely and appeared to be lost. He missed chiefly his three children. Both of us had our problems and we found comfort in being able to talk to each other, for both of us needed to piece our lives together again and, listening to his problems, somehow made mine easier to bear."

She sighed and went on, "Ralph and I soon became good friends and we even talked about getting engaged. Shortly afterwards, however, I missed a period. I discussed my fears with him but he didn't want to know and I soon realised that I meant nothing to him. I was at my wits ends. As week succeeded week I started to vomit and, fearing that I should die, I left the ship at the next port of call and flew to Paris where I entered an Abortion Clinic. They said I was ten weeks pregnant and that it was fortunate that I hadn't delayed any longer."

She paused to collect herself and then said, "I was still bleeding and had some pain when I awoke from the anaesthetic but they said that was normal and would continue for a few days. They gave me some panadol and sent me away. But I didn't get better. The pain and bleeding got worse and I thought I was going to die so I took the next flight to Heathrow and went and knocked up a friend who gave me a bed for the night." She would not let her friend contact her father so her friend, in desperation, drove her to the hospital where I was to work that day.

This tragic case indicates all too clearly that complications resulting from the ministrations of back street abortionists, which the 1967 Abortion Act was supposed to do away with, still occur from time to time in Government Licensed Abortion Clinics in Western countries. Abortion Clinics only care for their patients for the short time that it takes for the abortion to be performed and, unless a life-threatening incident occurs at that time, never see them again. It is left to the public or private hospital staff to deal with any complications that arise and all too frequently the cause of the complication does not feature in the published hospital statistics.

First of all we must ask what are the more common immediate complications of procured abortion? Obviously Sarah suffered from three of them, namely, perforation, haemorrhage, and infection, Perforation is said to occur in 2 to 3% of all terminations, and obviously, when dealing with a highly vascular pregnant uterus, perforation in these cases often results in haemor-rhage which, untreated may prove to be fatal. A further conse-quence of perforation, particularly if the abortionist is conscious that he/she has perforated the uterus and has wisely abstained from performing further suction curettage, is endometritis, that is the development of infection within the uterine cavity, due very often to the retention of products of conception (placental or foetal tissue). Such post-abortal infection is a risk for all women, and particularly for teenagers who are said to be 2.5 times more likely to develop infection than older women.

Pelvic inflammatory disease is another potentially life-threat-ening condition which can occur in women undergoing induced abortion and which can lead to an increased risk of subsequent ectopic pregnancy or infertility (an ectopic pregnancy is one occuring outside the uterus, most commonly in a uterine tube). It is particularly liable to occur in women who have a pre-existing chlamydial infection; indeed, it has been said that 23% of such patients will develop pelvic inflammatory disease within a month of their terminations.

Death, of course, still sometimes occurs following legal abor-tion. The main causes of such abortion related deaths are haem-orrhage, infection, embolism, anaesthesia and undiagnosed ectopic pregnancy. Indeed, in the United States Legal Abortion is reported to be the fifth leading cause of maternal death; and since it is recognised that most abortion related deaths are not official-ly reported as such it follows that it is probably much higher. Further more, the World Health Organization's coding of the Classification of Disease requires that deaths due to medical or surgical treatment are to be reported under the complication of the procedure rather than for the condition being treated, so this leads to further under-reporting of the primary condition.

Perhaps we should end by sparing a thought for the young lady whose life had been ruined. Did she become reconciled to her father? Did she enter University and complete her studies? Did she eventually marry and have a rewarding family life? All we can do is to hope that she, and others like her, were and are able to learn from their mistakes and make something out of their lives.

.

A Baby at any Cost

This case history is included because, although the only abortion that the patient had was a spontaneous one, it shows the other side of woman, namely those who prefer death itself to childlessness.

The journey to my Rooms took me through Regent's Park. It was early morning. The dew was on the grass but the morning sun was dispersing it and a slight vapour ascended to settle for a while on the pink blossom of the cherry trees before finally evaporating. I always relished this drive through the park for it usually afforded me the only opportunity I had to appreciate nature during my busy working week.

I should have liked to have stopped and to have walked round Queen Mary's Garden but time did not permit. I had a full clinic and my first patient was already waiting when I entered my Rooms. She was a 25-year-old Pakistani woman. Kausar looked sad and was quite pale. She had married six months previously and soon became pregnant. However, by the time she was 12 weeks pregnant her appearance suggested that she was almost double that size. An ultrasound had been performed and had revealed the presence of a large ovarian cyst containing both solid and fluid components. Laparotomy was performed and the right ovary, which contained a 20cm diameter cyst, was removed. Following this operation she unfortunately had a spontaneous abortion.

She handed me the operation report which indicated that the cyst was of borderline malignancy. Unfortunately no grading nor staging of the cyst's malignant potential had been carried out and her gynaecologist in Pakistan had recommended that the uterus and other ovary should be removed. This she had refused to consider so had come to London for a second opinion.

In London she had consulted a gynaecological oncologist who, to her chagrin, gave her the same advice. She told me that she wanted to be helped but also wished to retain her fertility. My clinical examination of her did not reveal an abnormality, and routine investigations that I carried out, which included a blood investigation for the ovarian cancer marker CA125 and Magnetic Resonance Imaging (MRI), were negative for cancer. I later understood that her husband was himself a trainee oncologist who had just obtained a training post at one of the London teaching hospitals. What were his views?

Kausar was an educated young lady. The position had been explained to her and the dilemma was that she could either run the risk of developing cancer or could lose any chance there was of having a baby. She sighed and said, "I had a happy childhood and joyful marriage and now this has happened. I'm not only mourning for the baby I've lost but am facing the prospect of never having another. I have a nightmare that my little ship will never again sail into the harbour of happiness." She looked tired and a tear rolled down her cheek.

I explained to her that there are many different types of ovarian cyst. "A borderline cyst," I said, "is not particularly dangerous. The trouble is we don't have all the information that we ought to have." She replied that because she had been pregnant her doctor wanted to do the minimum surgery that was necessary. She continued, "now that I've lost my baby I don't want to live if I'm unable to have children."

I was put in a quandary so I called in her husband in order that we could have a three-way discussion. It was finally agreed that further assessment was required. I explained that although preliminary investigations had been negative it would be necessary to perform further surgery to obtain biopsy specimens from the remaining ovary, lymph nodes, and the omentum (the fatty layer within the peritoneal cavity that hangs down like a curtain in front of the bowel) and to obtain peritoneal washings, so that the presence of malignant cells could be excluded before one could consider allowing her to become pregnant.

With permission granted I carried out laparoscopy, took peritoneal washings, used the Potassium-Titanyl-Phosphate (KTP) laser to separate the adhesions that had formed following the previous right ovariotomy (removal of the right ovary and the cyst within it), obtained several biopsies from lymph nodes, the remaining left ovary and omentum and finally arranged for my assistant to inject methylene blue dye through the cervix, and was happy to note that it flowed out freely through the uterine tubes and spilled into the peritoneal cavity, thus indicating that the uterine tubes had not been damaged by the previous operation and that, consequently, ova were capable of passing down the uterine tube in the opposite direction. All specimens were sent for histological examination and great was the rejoicing when no evidence of cancer was discovered.

In spite of the negative findings I was still a little nervous to allow Kausar to become pregnant so I made her wait for a further 12 months and then performed a second-look laparoscopy and took further washings and biopsy specimens. Only then when I again received negative results did I allow her to attempt to become pregnant.

She subsequently had three pregnancies and delivered three healthy babies. She was idyllically happy. Her husband, however, always carried the fear with him that she might, one day, develop cancer, but was somewhat reassured when I recommended that her other ovary should be removed once she had completed her family.

Borderline ovarian cancer is such an emotive subject that it is desirable to say a few words about it and to put it into perspective; for even Kausar with all the delight that she had in her children baulked at the prospect of being kept under observation and of the prospect that her other ovary would be removed once her family was complete. Although much research and information is available about borderline breast cancer little is known about borderline ovarian cancer. Patients want to know if they do or do not have ovarian cancer and the few patients whom I have treated for this condition and have kept under observation all suffered from a nagging doubt as to whether it might not be better to 'have everything out' and be done with it.

During each menstrual cycle a germ cell matures into an egg which is contained in a follicle or cyst, and this follicular cyst is covered with epithelium. Whilst maturation is proceeding the ovary produces oestrogen. When maturation is complete the follicle ruptures and the egg is released. The remnant of the follicular cyst is called a corpus luteum and is now responsible for the production of progesterone.

The epithelial covering of the follicular cyst may give rise to an ovarian cancer. Indeed, 80% of all ovarian cancers are epithelial in origin. They can be staged and consist of a spectrum of disease from benign cysts, through low-grade borderline cancers to stages I, II and III cancers. These cancers are often cystic and can rupture, disseminate their contents throughout the peritoneal cavity and adhere to the peritoneal surface, and hence to any organ which it contains.

In addition to stage the grade is also important. The lowest grade is designated 0. This refers to a low malignancy potential and is also called borderline cancer. Such cancers tend to be indolent and are diagnosed by their microscopic and histological appearance. They are expected to behave as very low-grade cancers. Some never become malignant while others may take fifteen or twenty years to develop.

Borderline ovarian cancers account for 10 to 20% of all ovarian tumours and are mainly diagnosed in young women. The most important features of malignant change are micro-invasion of the stroma and metastatic implants. Identification of those risk factors that indicate an adverse prognosis requires skilled interpretation by an experienced pathologist. Lack of proper information about Kausar's ovarian cyst made it difficult to decide what action it was best to take.

Guidelines for the surgical treatment of borderline ovarian tumours are similar to those of ovarian cancers and include laparotomy, peritoneal washings, hysterectomy and bilateral salpingo-oophorectomy (removal of both tubes and ovaries) or ovariotomy, omentectomy (excision of the fatty layer that hangs down in front of the bowel within the peritoneal cavity), multiple peritoneal biopsies and lymph node sampling.

Conservative surgery aimed at preserving childbearing potential is associated with a recurrence rate of 0 to 30 %. In Kausar's case we performed pelvic examination, trans-vaginal ultrasound, and CA125 measurements every three months for a year and then performed a second-look laparoscopy, together with peritoneal washings and further biopsies before allowing her to get pregnant. After that she remained under observation until she returned to Pakistan with her husband to whom I gave further instructions.

Research is still needed to follow up the psychological effect that such conservative treatment has on those patients. Certainly in this case it was great help to have Kausar's husband, himself an oncologist, to help in the decision making. Tailored counselling has been shown to be effective in helping to lessen distress and anxiety and in helping to sort out other problems, including those of a sexual nature.

The Anguish of Losing a Baby

E very day babies are stillborn or die shortly after birth and are labelled neonatal deaths. For these unfortunate mothers the suffering can be immense, so much so, indeed, that a society has been formed to help them to come to terms with their loss. However, little thought or compassion is spared for those women who lose their babies earlier in pregnancy, or whose eagerly expected baby turns out to be an ectopic one (a pregnancy developing outside the uterus, usually in one of the uterine tubes). Such women may suffer a similar amount of anguish but obtain little comfort by merely being told, "Don't worry. Twenty per cent of pregnancies end in abortion." There are those, too, with which this book is mainly concerned, who have chosen to have their pregnancies terminated and who later suffer pangs of remorse, or feelings of guilt, which may last for years, or, in some cases, for the whole of the rest of their lives.

This section or chapter deals with those women who, through no obvious fault of their own, suffer a first or second trimester abortion (miscarriage), and it consists, for the most part, of the uttered thoughts and musings of three of my patients who came to me for comfort after their sad ordeal.

Those who have experienced a stillbirth or neonatal death are devastated, but they do at least have an obstetrician, a midwife, and often a counsellor who, in some small measure, are able to sympathise and understand their sense of loss. Those who lose their baby earlier in pregnancy have the same feeling of devastation, but in some respects their suffering is greater. They were pregnant. They thought they had a baby but it was a chimera. There was nothing that they could feel or touch. They could not see it. There could be no memory. Their family and the hospital staff cannot quite understand their sense of loss. The woman herself cannot weep, and she has a feeling of dereliction. The comments of some of my patients can perhaps go a little way to explain the turmoil of soul which some of them experienced.

Sandra had a miscarriage when five months pregnant and came to see me to ask if I could find out why it had occurred. She told me that she had had a normal ultrasound scan and then, on the following day, her waters broke. She was admitted to hospital and kept there, but was told that the prognosis was poor. "Two weeks later", she said, "I miscarried when still less than 22 weeks pregnant." She continued, "The hospital staff were very kind and let my husband and me spend time with our little daughter so that we could say good bye to her in a dignified manner. Afterwards many people told me that it was very common to have a miscarriage, but nothing prepared me for the dreadful sense of loss that I experienced. We had been so excited when we knew that I was pregnant and we immediately started planning for her arrival." She paused, and then in a thoughtful frame of mind continued, "I remember, I was strolling in the park just a week before it happened. It was a wonderful day. The sky was brilliantly blue and the ground was dappled with spots of light from the sun that had filtered through the trees. I put my hand on my tummy and said, 'Dear little one, this is where I'm going to wheel you in the pram'."

She went on, "I looked up. The air was motionless, but when I opened my mouth to breath I noticed a faint chill, like the chill you notice when you first take up a glass of iced water before you take a sip. I continued walking in the park and breathing deeply to give more fresh air to my baby. How could I know that it was all to no avail?"

She was silent for a short time and then said, "How could all my hopes be turned to dust and ashes? When I started to produce milk for a baby that was no longer there it was unbearable! How can any one understand what it's like to grieve for a baby who's not there?"

She wanted me to carry out a thorough investigation to determine what was the cause of her miscarriage, for she just could not face a similar tragedy occurring again. This I did and discovered that she had an incompetent cervix.

In fullness of time she again became pregnant and I encircled her cervix with a stitch. On this occasion, although remaining very apprehensive throughout, she carried her pregnancy to term and I delivered her of a healthy little girl. Although delighted with her new baby she said that she could never forget the ordeal that she went through with her first baby whom she continued to call, Helena. She also insisted that her new baby was not a replacement for Helena. She was a completely new individual.

Knowing that I had at one stage told her that, when I had time, I was going to write a book for women who had had terminations of pregnancy, she said, "The trauma of miscarriage and the subsequent grieving that occurs afterwards is quite as bad as is that experienced by women who have had terminations"; and she asked me to include something of what she had told me when I came to write the book.

Another of my patients, Caroline by name, who, in fact, had been pro-choice, said that losing your baby meant losing a part of yourself. She continued, "It means losing your dreams, not your own private dreams, but dreams involving your family life."

At the beginning of her marriage, three years before, she had a termination, but this latter one had been planned, was much wanted, but turned out to be an ectopic pregnancy.

She said, "Sometimes you may not be aware of all those dreams until you know that the baby is irrevocably gone. We were happily married, had planned everything, and when the right moment arrived I became pregnant. We had even decorated baby's room before I conceived."

Continuing she said, "After the ectopic pregnancy had been diagnosed and I was fighting for my life and later recovering from the operation, it was then that it hit me. Nobody prepares you for this possibility when you are pregnant. You're looking forward to starting a family and then all your hopes are taken away. The most difficult thing about this raw grief is the question, 'Why did it happen?'"

She went on, "Another factor is isolation. Expressions of grief are so taboo in our society that sometimes it's hard to grieve properly. You feel that no one understands and no one cares." Finally she posed this question, "Why should you feel sad when the baby isn't even a person yet?"

Carmen was a 35-year-old bright, young lady in a well-established general practitioner practice. She was ambitious, worked hard, and also managed to care for two young children. She had not planned another pregnancy, but when she found that she was pregnant, she was delighted, reorganized her working life and began to look forward to the arrival of the newcomer. She and her husband arranged for an extra room to be built and even helped to paint and decorate it in preparation for the new arrival.

When she was 20 weeks pregnant her legs became swollen and she no longer felt the delicate movements that she had experienced during the preceding two weeks. She went to the hospital and the obstetrician, after listening said, "I'm afraid I can't hear a heart beat."

Carmen was annoyed at the doctor's remark. She did not believe it, or rather, she did not want to believe it. An ultrasound was arranged. Carmen was very frightened. She did not want to face reality. "I could not face the reality that baby was dead," she explained, "the reality that someone was going to take the baby away. I held my abdomen with both my hands. But then all my hopes will be taken away from me. It's best not to know!"

The ultrasound nevertheless took place and the doctor

frowned and said, "I'm afraid there's no heart beat." "No heart beat?" I murmured, "It was repeated in my mind. Suddenly you are mourning the loss of your bright future and all the rites of passage that you now wont be able to experience, from baby's first bath to his first birthday party. Perhaps the most difficult aspect of such grief is that there may be no answer to the question, 'Why?'"

She told me that she left the hospital and went home to cry. Although she knew that the baby was dead she did not want any interference, just in case he was alive. She still wanted to believe that he was. She lay awake in bed trying to pray but being quite unable to focus her thoughts.

She said, "the radiologist's words kept pounding in my head, 'There's no heart beat. There's no heart beat.' I felt I couldn't breath. My heart was tight, as though bound with chains. All night long I lay awake while myriads of conflicting thoughts assailed my brain. Eventually I went into labour and delivered a beautiful little boy, but he was still-born. For months I suffered feelings of failure and anger. I felt cheated and robbed of my child."

I looked at her with a feeling of compassion. Battered, trembling, yet still proud, I sensed the anguish and feeling of desolation that she suffered. After a momentary pause she continued, "After I had painted his room and had prepared all his furniture I started to cough. That's really why I went to hospital. I didn't want anyone to check my baby. I sometimes felt that I couldn't breath. At other times I thought my heart had stopped beating and that I had fallen into a black hole from which there was no escape."

Changing her train of thought Carmen continued, "I also struggled with feelings of guilt. Did the paint and varnish fumes poison the baby? Was it something that I had eaten? Had I been working too hard? Had pollution in the air affected me? Question after question kept assailing me. I desperately wanted the heartache to become a soft, sad memory, not a bitter part of every day life."

She further said, "If I were not a doctor I would see a counsellor, but I cannot. I must be strong. My husband is a Paediatrician looking after sick babies, but our baby is dead and for which no obvious cause can be found. At times I was even cross with God. Why had he taken an innocent life of one who had not even had a chance to enjoy some of it? I came to realise that I was not only mourning for a child, but also for the dreams that went with it. I had seen the chid but not his smile, and I had not participated in his play.

She again said, "I really feel guilty." "Guilty of what?" I enquired. "What is the Charge?" The fact was she had not accepted that her child had died inside. "Was that such a crime?" I asked. "Was it a crime to go on hoping? What mother wants to believe that her child has died?" Carmen replied, "I really can't forget that beautiful face. As a medical practitioner she can really only understand the emotion and anguish that a patient experiences when she has a stillbirth or loses a child, when in fact she has a similar experience herself.

She finally said, "It would be good to write something down about this catastrophe. In medical school we all learn about the symptoms and signs of miscarriage, abortion, ectopic pregnancy, stillbirth, neonatal death and even cot death, and how to deal with them. However, none of us is equipped to deal with the real life emotions of a patient who has lost her child, nor of the emotional trauma, which may remain with the woman for years to come. One recovers from the physical side of the miscarriage or delivery, the feelings of guilt, failure, and anger slowly pass, but the feelings of grief and emptiness remain for years. For at least a year after I lost my baby I would find myself crying when I drove to work. Although I was busy at work and at home, where I also had my living children to attend, I, nevertheless, felt sad for most of the time. What right had I to feel sad when it wasn't as though I had lost a real child? Was it?"

This last patient was speaking sarcastically for she was fully aware that she had lost a precious baby. It might be helpful, therefore, to say a little about spontaneous abortion:

Most people associate the word 'abortion' with termination of pregnancy, but doctors also use the same word to describe miscarriage, which can be defined as the ending of a pregnancy due to premature delivery before the baby is able to survive outside the uterus.Nowadays it is defined as occurring before 20 completed weeks of gestation, or, according to the World Health Organization, if it weighs less than 500gm. After that it is termed a premature birth, or, if born dead, it is called a still birth.

In past ages it was always considered that the woman was at fault if she miscarried, but it is now known that in many cases the father's sperm is defective.Thus, older men have older spermatozoa that can contribute to theproduction of defective zygotes (fertilized eggs), a common cause of miscarriage. Similarly smoking, drinking and taking of proscribed drugs by either partner can have the same deleterious effect. About half of all early miscarriages occur because of the way in which the genetic material from the egg and sperm have combined during fertilization.

Other causes of miscariage are hormonal inbalance, problems with the immune system, and certain infections; while uterine malformations, uterine fibroids (benign uterine tumours) or cervical weakness or incompetence may also be responsible.

Much could be written about spontaneous abortion, which acounts for foetal loss in some 20% of pregnancies. What matters, however, is that loss of a baby is an emotional and traumatic event in a woman's life that has been greatly underestimated by medical practitioners and, indeed, by society in general. Great understanding and compassion are required to manage these women with kindness and with efficiency.

Custom and Tradition

Mrs Ho was a modern, well-educated Chinese woman of 25 years of age married to a successful, rich, Westernized Chinese businessman some six years older than herself. Having successfully negotiated the perils and pitfalls of their early business life together they had now to embarked on the more mundane, but equally important, task of producing an heir for the family fortune.

Mrs Ho had decided to have her baby privately with me and had faithfully attended for antenatal care. I had performed an early ultrasound examination to confirm that she was pregnant and that it was contained within the uterus, and now that she had reached the sixteenth week of pregnancy she had come with her husband to have a further ultrasound examination to confirm that the pregnancy was progressing normally. They appeared to be a loving couple and it was a pleasure to see that the husband took so much interest in his wife's progress.

Having prepared the ultrasound machine and positioned Mrs Ho appropriately on the examination couch I called in the husband so that they could both view the screen and see their baby. He gently laid aside his coat and slowly made his way over to the couch to be near his wife. Having often seen businessmen in my rooms who were nearly always in a hurry it was a joy to meet one who obviously cared for his wife and wished to share in her enjoyment. They had great delight in seeing the baby sucking its thumb and then jigging up and down as though on a trampoline. Yes, this was what they had been waiting for. Her husband smiled and, looking round at his wife and then again at the ultrasound picture, he laughed and said, "I love that little boy." They both became silent and a cloud seemed to settle on the two. I was surprised so, to break the tension, I said, "Baby looks healthy. That's why we're doing the ultrasound to confirm that it is so. Indeed that's why we do ante-natal care to ensure, as far as possible, that a healthy baby is eventually born."

"By the way, what is the baby's sex, doctor?" the husband suddenly asked. Before I could answer Mrs Ho interrupted and said, "Don't ask that question, dear. I don't want to know. It's much better if it's a surprise." She faltered and again became silent. The husband appeared to be annoyed. He put on his coat and left the examination room. I could not imagine what was troubling them for they both appeared to be distressed at what should have been a most joyful occasion.

When Mrs Ho had dressed she returned to my consulting room and I noticed that a tear was rolling down her cheek. She said, "I hope it's a boy. My husband would like to have a son." I replied, "Well, the important thing is that the baby's healthy, and this seems to be the case." She gave a sickly smile and replied, "Of course." Something still seemed to be bothering her but I thought that perhaps she was apprehensive because it was her first baby. I asked her if she had family and friends in this country, and when she replied that she had, I felt more relieved to know that there would be those to help and guide her through her pregnancy.

The antenatal period was uneventful. Sometimes her husband accompanied her when she came to visit me and sometimes she came alone. Finally she went into labour and I delivered her of a healthy little girl. Her husband could not be present, but all of us who were in the delivery suit were delighted.

The following morning when I visited Mrs Ho in hospital she looked withdrawn and withered, even distraught. There were no flowers on her bedside locker and no baby in a cot beside her. I asked the midwife the reason for the latter and she told me that Mrs Ho had asked that the baby should be cared for in the nursery. I thought at first that she must be suffering from postnatal depression, but that seemed to be most unlikely. I therefore settled myself down in a chair at her bedside, took her hand in mine, and asked her what the trouble was.

She hesitatingly began to tell me the whole story. It appeared that although they were Westernized old customs from their nation's past still survived, and one was the importance of having a male heir. Had her husband known that it would be a daughter he would have insisted that it should be aborted. She however could not face that possibility. She had now disgraced her husband and family by having given birth to a female child. No one would visit her, not even her husband, and she seemed to be completely ostracized. Her husband, indeed, had upbraided her for not having obtained the sex of the foetus. Had he known what the outcome would be he would have insisted that it should be aborted, for essentially abortion on demand is permitted in the West; whereas had they still been in China, although the sex of the child might not have been known before birth, nevertheless infanticide could then have been performed. In this country, however, that is not allowed.

I was so disturbed by Mrs Ho's heartrending account of her trouble that I took advantage of the forthcoming weekend to spend a day at the seaside to think through and to try to make sense of it all.

I got up very early on the following morning, indeed before the sun had risen, and so arrived at my destination when the morning was still young. Behind me were the Downs with their lush grass, scattered stunted trees and flocks of sheep, while ahead was the grey sea, for the sun was still low in the sky but strong enough to be slowly dispersing the mist. The ground was wet with dew and the fuchsias and nasturtiums were covered with droplets of water. It was good, too, to smell the damp earth again after so long tramping the hard pavements of London.

Approaching the promenade I listened with delight to the gentle rustle and plashing of the sea. I was passed by a gentleman walking his old dog who cut a caper or two, but who then drew up as if ashamed of his levity, and then walked a few dignified paces at his master's side once again.

My mind reverted to Mrs Ho. Was there anything that I could do to help her in her distress? I could not accept the old Chinese custom of abortion on account of the sex of the foetus, but what about the West's ability now to obtain an abortion on any sex merely by request? Why should that be any more acceptable than the Chinese custom of sex discrimination, either achieved by abortion or by infanticide at birth?

East and West are both guilty and judicial murder has even been carried out for the same purpose; so I let my mind dwell for a moment on the unfortunate Anne Boleyn who was beheaded on a trumped up charge of adultery because she could not provide King Henry VIII with a live male heir. Illogical as it was Mrs Ho, in her husband and family's eyes, was just as guilty. Tradition told them that it was so and Mrs Ho recognised this and was depressed, ashamed, even guilty. This was a recognition of her national consciousness, even though she had abandoned her country and was living in an entirely different environment. It was certainly not post-natal depression. Even with today's mass migration people shape their lives and behaviour by the way they are brought up.

I stumbled over a stone, awoke from my reverie and looked about. The sun now shone forth in all his glory and the mist had fled away, vanished. The sky, previously a pale grey but now a clear bright blue, was reflected in the puddles, and more particularly in the sea itself, which danced and threw up little white bursts of spray and spindrift. The brightness of God's creation made my eyes ache to look at it.

My thoughts kept escaping from me and I wished as a doctor that we could do more to help our patients. "Perhaps in many cases," I mused, "the best we can do is to be a patient and sympathetic listener, not an easy task in this present frenetic life that we live. How can we ignore the thousands of years of custom and tradition?"

As I was meditating on these things the morning breeze freshened and made me once again conscious of the good, black, wet soil, which for a moment displaced the salty tang of the sea. Myriads of birds were singing a song of praise to their Maker and I again thought of the man whom I had seen walking his dog. In England it is said that man's best friend is his dog, whereas in some cultures dogs are considered unclean and are not tolerated anywhere near human habitation. Thus, throughout the centuries cultures have passed on their national and family values to succeeding generations. Our opinions are shaped by traditions and rituals, while repetitive practice of customs become unwritten law and regulate our social life.

Suddenly a lady approached followed by a Dalmatian dog. She did not have him on a lead. Instead she called to him and he obediently followed her. Recognizing that she was Scottish I remembered that when I had attended a medical congress in Scotland the Scots had, on one particular day, celebrated some national event that appeared to be steeped in tradition. Many were wearing the kilt, the different clans or tribes wore their distinctive tartan and their ceremonial was accompanied by the skirl of the bagpipes. By those rituals they proclaimed loyalty to their nation whose beginnings were lost in the obscurity of pre-written history.

All nations have customs or traditions and some, indeed, pass from nation to nation. One of the oldest relates to the launching of ships. The most ancient so far discovered was carved on an Assyrian stone tablet in about 2,100 BC. It records the launching of Noah's Ark and notes that a yoke of oxen were sacrificed when the Ark was launched. Similarly Fijians and Samoans made human sacrifice to the sharks, whom they thought of as gods, and washed their canoes with the sacrificial blood when they were launched. Legend too tells how the Vikings launched their ships of war over the bodies of young men who were crushed to death by the keels during the launching ceremony. Nowadays, of course, the ritual is replaced by a bottle of Champaign or wine being broken against the side of the ship.

Those traditions encouraging the cooperation and wellbeing of the nation, or that are of a celebratory character, should be retained, while those of a harmful or superstitious nature are best abandoned, particularly when they harm or damage innocent victims. As an obstetrician my task was to deliver my patient of a healthy baby who should bring joy and happiness to both the mother and her husband.

It is obvious that those cultures and customs, which remain the same at every period of a nation's history, respond to the permanent needs of the people. We are not concerned here about individual differences. Education should evoke our humanity and not simply develop our individuality. Surely humanity and the power of reasoning are those things that distinguish us from all other animals.

The offering of the life of a human being to a god in some ancient cultures was an attempt to communicate with the god and to participate in the divine life. Nowadays we marvel at such a misunderstanding. I wonder how we shall be judged by future generations for destroying our own offspring,

Resentment

In our journey through India we reached a small village near the lake in the middle of which was a Maharana's palace, now converted into a luxury hotel, and made famous by James Bond's film, "Octopussy". I contrasted the opulence of this palace in Udaipur with the mud hovels that I now encountered. No roads, no streets, no gardens; filth everywhere with a few chicken picking amidst the garbage. Yet amazingly the people appeared to be contented. Women sat at their doors to watch their ragged or naked children playing in the dust, while the old men, one without a hand, another without a leg, also sat immobile but in quiet converse.

The appearance of foreigners in their midst led to immediate activity. Soon we were surrounded by beggars, with children to the fore, asking for money. We scattered a few rupees and smaller coins that we had to the throng and with this they were well content. Perhaps the most grateful was a man who had no arms at all but who received a piece of paper money in his mouth.

I considered this amazing sub-continent where untold wealth rubbed shoulders with abject poverty and wondered what had prevented it from erupting into civil war and bloodshed. It must surely be the Hindu religion and philosophy. Many of their priests and gurus led Spartan lives, so it would seem that the poor did not consider their lot to be anything out of the ordinary. Previously in Bombay, or Mombai as it is now called, we had visited a Jain temple on Malabar Hill where we had seen devotees wearing masks and sweeping the floor to avoid damaging or crushing any of the insects,

Passing on from this nameless village we soon entered the city of Udaipur where hovels gave way to expensive residences, soon to be followed by the palace of Udai Sing which stands on a ridge overlooking the lake. Nevertheless, although this massive structure with its striking roof gardens was impressive enough, my eyes were instinctively drawn to the smaller Jag Nivas palace, situated on an island in the centre of the lake which was to be the hotel in which we were to stay. Built in 1622 as a pleasure palace for imperial parties and functions it served as a shelter for Shahjahan against the wrath of his father, the Mogul Emperor Jahangir, for refusing to take charge of an expedition to retake Qandahar that had been recently recaptured by the energetic king of Persia, Shah Abbas. Shahjahan, it will be remembered, was the one who later commissioned the building of the Taj Mahal on the banks of the Jumna River in Agra as a fitting memorial and mausoleum for his beloved wife, Mumtaz. Shahjahan had originally planned to build a black mausoleum for himself on the other side of the Jumna linking it by bridge, but his son had other ideas and locked him up in prison where he spent the remainder of his days; similar, I thought, to the way many children in the West put their old parents in Care Homes.

Arriving at the landing stage we were taken across to the palace in a boat where we were met by a hotel official that allocated a room to us but told our Indian friend who had accompanied us that he could not be accommodated in the palace but would need to find accommodation ashore. It would seem that the Palace, which having fallen on hard times, was eventually give a new lease of life by being turned into a luxury hotel exclusively for the use of foreigners, a kind of apartheid in reverse.

Having bade farewell to our Indian friend we seated ourselves in the lobby while our room was prepared for us and watched the other guests who were milling around. There, for instance, was an old South American gentleman speaking quietly in Spanish to a striking young woman in a red dress. On the other side of the room were three little Japanese men in dark suits conferring discreetly together, quite inappropriately dressed, I thought, for such a hot climate. In another part of the room I caught a glimpse of a very famous American Film Director. Letting my eyes wander further they alighted on an Arab Sheik with some eight body-guards and three wives. Finally I caught a glimpse of several young men in lightweight suits, probably American, who were conversing with a very beautiful, self-contained young woman wearing a sky-blue Channel linen suit.

The porter took our cases to our room which we found to be modest in size but with the white marble walls inlaid with most beautiful jewel-like flowers of coloured glass. Once again I compared this fairy-like sumptuous apartment, and, indeed, the whole lavish splendour of the palace with its white marble floors and inlaid walls of coloured glass in designs of lotus and leaf patterns, which, even so, must have been a shadow of its former glory with its marble piazzas enclosing orange trees, cypresses and loft palm trees, with the abject poverty almost visible across the lake.

Returning to one of the public rooms I found the lady in the blue suit sitting by herself near a window. I wanted to ask her if they were filming in the hotel so I took a seat nearby and we soon struck up an acquaintance. To my question about the filming she replied that she did not know, so it soon became apparent that she was not connected with the other Americans whom I had previously seen. I then went on to comment on the poverty but apparent contentment of the Indian lower classes, in spite of the great wealth which often surrounded them. "I detest their contentment," she replied. "They do nothing at all to better themselves." She went on to say, "I'm working at full speed and wonder sometimes how I can keep going. Even when my body is quivering from weariness and cries out for rest I keep on and on, for all too easily the dread memories come creeping back." "Work," she said, is the only thing that keeps me from thinking. I've been told that there are healers in this country, and this is why I've come. My whole life revolves round my life's work and its success. Perhaps one day it will satisfy my soul's craving, but it hasn't done so yet." She then abruptly changed her train of thought and added, "I detest those ignorant villagers who are satisfied with the little they have!"

I was amazed at her outburst and by the way she unburdened her heart to a complete stranger. I wondered if there was some deep-seated problem in her life that had soured her relationships with her fellow men. I asked if she had any children. "No!" she indignantly replied, "I had a termination when I first became pregnant. Thank God I'm free from all that; but I work very hard. I don't know anything about the wind, or the sky, or the trees until I go on holiday, and even this is a working holiday. I don't enjoy any time that I do have free. I have a constant longing for I don't know what. I just have to keep going."

My husband joined me at that moment so I had no further talk with her that night. What was the cause of this woman's distress? Was she secretly envious of the poor people around with their pitifully small belongings and their growing families? Undoubtedly she was in desperate need of some counselling, and it surprised me that she did not have her own psychiatrist or psychoanalyst. Or had she tried them and found them wanting?

The following morning I saw Jane again in the breakfast room. It was seven o'clock but she was already tucking into substantial fare. "Hi there", she said. She sounded bright and alert and was already in a hurry. "What are you doing today?" I enquired. "I have a business meeting. Then my business partner will be taking me to a clothing factory." She smiled and continued, "There at least the children are employed and work for very little money. I'm considering transferring my business here, for I've calculated that once it's up and running it will cost me ten times less than it would back home." That was the last I was to see of Jane but the question kept on going round in my head as to why she had had an abortion and why she appeared to dislike children so much, except when they could be exploited. I wondered too whether she really was going to look for a healer or guru to help her. I thought it was most unlikely unless she had a nervous breakdown.

My husband and I had arranged to meet that morning our Indian friend who was to take us to the north of Udaipur to visit some temples, including Eklingji, one of the prime pilgrimage destinations of Hindu devotees of Lord Siva in Rajasthan. As in the case with most temples in this region the shrine is built of white marble, but it houses a large, four-faced black marble image of Siva. Now although Siva, the third of the Hindu trinity, is the Destroyer, nevertheless he is also worshipped as the god of fertility, medicine and physical love, and so has many zealous followers. Outside the main shrine, besides a stone statue of Nandi, Siva's bull-mount, one came across several small stone Linga. It is interesting to realise that throughout India Siva is worshipped through Lingam (the phallus) and consequently Linga in stone are more common than statues of Siva. The worship of a fertility god or goddess, has occurred for thousands of years in most parts of the world. To mention just a few: Bast the cat-headed goddess of Ancient Egypt, Mylitta the Assyrian and Babylonian goddess, Baal the Canaan god, Aphrodite of ancient Greece, Mars a Roman fertility god (besides being the god of war), Frigg the wife of Odin, Kokopelli a native American fertility god. Finally, to revert to the temple of Eklingji and to complete the picture, it is worth notin g that its name is derived from Ek meaning one and ling meaning the life-giving phallic symbol of Lord Siva.

These thoughts all took me back to Jane and her apparent abhorrence of children and child bearing, except insofar as they could be exploited. In India and in most countries in the East, with a few exceptions amongst the wealthy, the people had children as a form of security for the future and with the knowledge that they will look after them in their old age. In the secular West however 'consumerism' has become all-important. Fewer children are being born, more are being aborted and the young have followed fashion by putting their old 'disposable' parents into old people's care homes, usually against their mothers and fathers wishes or desires. It is frightening to think that euthanasia might well be their next line of attack!

The Abortionist's Story

P eter is a composite character. In my years of medical practice I met a number of doctors whose primary aim changed from that of being a healer of the sick to one of intent on the acquisition of wealth. And what better way to achieve that quickly than by working in an Abortion Clinic, and even becoming the director or, if possible, the owner of that establishment? And should that occupation begin to pall then one could always direct an In Vitro Fertilization Centre which depends so largely upon treating patients whose infertility problems are often the result of complications that have followed previous terminations.

Not all, of course, spend their whole lives in the abortion scene. A few have concluded that what they have been doing is wrong, and some have written frankly about their change of heart.

In my time in medicine I have had dealings with some of those doctors. They represent one facet that needs to be examined if we are to explore the whole abortion controversy. I have linked together meetings that I had with three of those medical colleagues to make a story that hangs together, and which also examines their philosophy. This is not to say that there are not a few doctors who altruistically believe that what they are doing is for the good of mankind, but, if so, they must be an extremely small minority:

As I learnt later, Peter was a bright young man who had done well at medical school and who, during the transition between his pre-clinical and clinical studies, had spent two months in France honing his knowledge of the French language. Handsome, eloquent and popular, he had no shortage of lady friends.

Following graduation he spent his pre-registration year working in the National Health Service as a Houseman, but soon realized that he could not tolerate the hard grind and subservience required to succeed in the profession he had chosen. He had drive, ambition, and certain entrepreneurial skills, and confessed that he had chosen medicine as a way, he had mistakenly thought, to wealth and fame. He entered the pharmaceutical industry; was very successful in marketing drugs, and was soon earning four times as much as he had done as a young doctor in the NHS.

He married Mary, a bright, final year medical student, who had decided to enter general practice. Mary too, was ambitious. She had had a steady boyfriend, a fellow medical student who was loving and kind, but noting how successful Peter had become, she changed her allegiance, and was soon engaged and later married to him.

Peter progressed from strength to strength and became a manager. However, he was not content to remain a player in someone else's company, so having learnt all he could regarding business and marketing, he left the company, branched out in a different direction, and set up a private abortion clinic.

When I was still a very young doctor I saw an advertisement in a medical journal offering £500 for an afternoon's work in a clinic each week. It did not specify the type of work required so I was intrigued. Such a job would allow me plenty of time to study medicine until I threw myself, once again, into the hurly-burly of another medical appointment. I rang the telephone number provided to enquire about the work that was required to be carried out in the clinic and was told that it consisted of performing some twenty abortions during an afternoon's session! How could I accept? I wanted a job to help me to improve my knowledge of how to save life, not to destroy it. I said that I was not interested.

The following day, when I was sitting in a gloomy hospital library looking at a medical textbook, a good-looking, impeccably dressed young man bounced in. It was Peter. He not only worked in the clinic that I had phoned, but actually owned it. His intention, it appeared, was to induce me to reconsider my refusal. He laughed at my simplicity, or as he considered it, my stupidity. How was it, he inquired, that I was prepared to work night and day in a dismal hospital and was not even prepared to give his job a try? He had his own helicopter, was looking to expand his clinic, and was particularly anxious to employ a young lady doctor. As a further inducement he said that if I were prepared to become a partner I would earn more than ten times my NHS salary.

I attempted to argue with him, and said what I had thought on the previous day, namely, that my aim was to save life and not to destroy it. He replied that most abortions dealt with foetal abnormalities. He continued, "Disabled people suffer and no one can help them. Their quality of life is very poor and they are a burden to their families and on society." He continued to use his charm and said, "If all the money saved on caring for the disabled was used for the poor and disadvantaged, think what better quality of life the people in the world would have?"

Peter was older than I and much more experienced and skillful in argument. Indeed, he was not really interested at all in my reasoning. Like all marketing experts his aim was to convince the listener of the rightness of his conclusions, and to overcome any doubts that the listener might have. He was not interested at all in a two-way discussion.

He said, "You're a woman. You should be on the same side as women. Desperately poor women can't cope with more children. They've struggled for years to have the Abortion Law altered. You should be trying to help them."

By this time Peter realised that he could not tempt me by offering a huge salary, so he change tack. Accepting my contention that I wanted to save lives he said, "Don't you know that women suffer, and often die, from the attentions of back street abortionists?" He then showed me some mortality and morbidity statistics attributed to such illegal operations, and continued, "If you joined me you could certainly save the lives of those women." I queried, "What about the lives of the unborn?" Realising that he was not going to make a convert of me, he finally said, "We do abortions when there are foetal abnormalities, or if children are unwanted. We want a world in which women have complete freedom; a world free from disabled and unwanted children!"

Many years later I met Peter again, this time at a Medical Congress in Paris. In spite of our different outlooks on life Peter remained sociable and friendly. He asked me back for tea in his hotel. Ordering a taxi he spoke in impeccable French, and everything he did and said suggested that he was in command and a man of impressive stature. It was obvious that there was much more to him than his well-tailored bespoke suit, his starched white shirt, and his expensive briefcase.

Peter was staying at the Ritz so while he paid the driver I gazed at the nearby host of impressive shops. He had chosen a hotel which reeked of decadent luxury, for it offered its patrons unlimited comfort. As he stepped through the revolving doors one could sense that he felt a tinge of excitement. The subtle elegance and exquisite décor gratified his appetite for beauty.

Peter ordered tea and it appeared that he still wanted to prove to me that he was right. It seemed that he believed that his expensive hotel showed that to be the case. I was staying at a more modest establishment and said that although I liked his hotel very much I could not afford to stay there.

We sat over tea and gave each other our news. Peter told me that everything had been going very well until the law had changed regarding late abortions. He himself claimed to be an expert in late abortions. Their necessity was, he declared, usually occasioned by the finding of foetal abnormalities that had not been detected earlier in the pregnancy. "Parliament," he said, "has no business to interfere with the rights of women to do whatever they wish with their own bodies, even if they are eight and a half months pregnant. It is quite immoral to see a twenty-six week old alien thing hooked up to tubes and wires, and fighting for its life in an incubator."

After the law had been modified his clinic had become a focus for opposition. Bomb threats were made, the clinic had to be evacuated, and staff and patients were herded, shivering onto the pavement outside, while sniffer dogs explored the evacuated building. On another occasion people broke in, stole files and destroyed equipment, while on a still further occasion someone broke in early in the morning and poured fuel oil all over the floor. Fortunately he was disturbed before he could set it alight. Although no shots were ever fired at them, nevertheless, it was thought wise to install bullet-proof glass in the windows and to hire security guards to patrol the building and keep protestors away from patients entering the clinic. Rain or shine, protesters were outside, shouting, singing, and holding placards depicting pictures of aborted babies and foetal remains, with some even being graphically laid out and displayed on white towels. They came early and left late.

Life had become so difficult, he told me, for himself and his staff that he was planning to move and set up somewhere else. That, indeed, was why he had come to Paris, for he wished to explore all possibilities.

He still wondered if I had changed my mind and whether I was impressed by his luxurious lifestyle. Would I not, even at this late stage, like to throw in my lot with him? I told him that I had trained in minimally invasive laser surgery in gynaecology and had been impressed by observing what had already been achieved by certain laser surgeons, using such methods, to correct a few foetal abnormalities in utero.

I told him that I had been involved in some research on foetal calves while still within the uterus. I had used open surgery and similar operations had, since then, also been carried out in other centres. More recently, however, I explained that the foetoscope had been used in humans, and now certain malformations could be dealt with while the foetus was still within the mother's uterus, such as the closure of a congenital diaphragmatic hernia (a deficiency in part of the diaphragm that allows part of the stomach , small intestine or colon to pass into the thoracic cavity) or the resection of a cystadenomatoid malformation of the lung (a cystic malformation of part of the lung).

Peter stopped me and said that the medical profession was repeatedly being faced with ethical dilemmas throughout its working life. It had to decide how best to service resources, and how time, money, and skills could best be apportioned. In particular, he suggested that medical scientific advances were outstripping the nation's ability to fund them.

I replied that it was our duty, as doctors, to do our best with the facilities available, not only to save lives, but to ensure that the lives thus saved were of sterling quality. I told him that many conditions could now be treated by laser, employing a minimally invasive approach. Endoscopic visualization of the foetus after nearly half a century was now advanced and surgical procedures were now being successfully carried out. "For instance," I continued, "surgical treatment of babies with cleft lip and cleft palate, although successful, tended to leave unsightly scars, whereas now, if performed on the foetus in utero, not only is the operation successful, but the operation leaves a scarless result."

I said that my experience in animal research had shown that foetal wound healing and repair was quite different from that observed in postnatal life. The change over from foetal to postnatal type of healing occurred late in its gestation stage. The foetal healing and repair process was characterized by the absence of an inflammatory reaction. The intracellular matrix had a very high content of hyaluronic acid which accelerated cell migration and regeneration, with the result that wound contracture did not occur. Those and other processes ensured that, in prenatal life, wound healing occurred without scar formation.

Peter by this time looked more subdued. He agreed that some abnormalities were amenable to treatment but that many more still could not be treated by intra-uterine surgery. I had to agree with him and said that much more research was still needed. Peter, ever resourceful to make his point of view known, said that some abnormalities were, even at this time, not detected in early pregnancy; that some teenagers did not realize that they were pregnant; and that, therefore, there was still a need for some late abortions. I thus saw that Peter was once again trying to justify his actions.

My final meeting with Peter occurred a few years later when I met him, quite unexpectedly, in Sydney, Australia. He had apparently made his way there to further his career. The previous year, however, he had been involved in a serious car accident and had barely escaped with his life. Many of the bones in his body had been broken, and it was obvious that his legs would never be the same again.

I met him being pushed by Mary, his wife, in a wheel chair. She was working as a general practitioner, and he himself was endeavouring to assist her in her surgery. How his life had changed! He complained that most public places were not organized to accommodate the disabled, and he had been thinking how things might be improved. Indeed, he had campaigned for the rights of the disabled.

Peter had changed, not only in physical appearance, but also within. He was still as intelligent as before, but was no longer obsessed by the love of money. He had developed a compassion for the physically and mentally disadvantaged, and our whole conversation was centred around those topics.

As it was nearly lunchtime I suggested that he and his wife should be my guest. He gratefully accepted my invitation. His wife settled him at the table in his wheel chair, and I noted with sadness, that on account of his twisted face, food sometimes dribbled out of his mouth and fell on his napkin. To save embarrassing him I turned my face away and at that moment remembered Shakespeare's Macbeth soliloquy:

> Tomorrow, and tomorrow, and tomorrow,
> Creeps in this petty pace from day to day
> To the last syllable of recorded time;
> And all our yesterdays have lighted fools
> The way to dusty death. Out, out brief candle!
> Life's but a walking shadow, a poor player
> That struts and frets his hour upon the stage
> And then is heard no more; it is a tale
> Told by an idiot, full of sound and fury,
> Signifying nothing.

He appeared now to be more kind and compassionate, no longer concerned only with his own happiness. He confessed that he had been wrong to think that by aborting abnormal babies one could eliminate disability from the world. He said that there were so many like him who had been injured, not only in car accidents, but also in war and by natural disasters. All one could do was to make their lives as comfortable as possible.

I agreed, but said that society had progressed considerably from the days when people with disabilities were feared and therefore discriminated against. One only had to read history or some novels of a century or so ago, to understand how the sinister hump of Richard III, the evil prosthesis of Captain Hook, or the thumping wooden leg of Captain Ahab instilled fear into those who came into contact with them.

I suggested that International Human Rights' treaties played an important role in protecting the rights of people with disabilities. Peter reiterated the fact that he had been active in the human rights movement in Australia. He sighed and said that, although he was pleased with progress much still remained to be done.

Although I was sorry for Peter in the condition in which I found him, nevertheless, after talking to him I realized that he was a changed man. His view of life had profoundly altered, and I was impressed by the voluntary work that he was doing and by his compassion and concern for those in need. He was not the first doctor whom I had met who had changed from being an abortionist to becoming a saint.

Peter remained silent for a few minutes and gazed at the floor. He was plucking up courage to unburden his soul to me. Eventually he said, "We have had disagreements in the past. I used to be young and strong and believed that all the world should be like that. I was wrong. In my stiff-necked rebellion I thought that all imperfect things should be erased, and I did my best to see that they were. Divine justice, however, pursued me. Disasters came thick and fast until, finally, I was almost destroyed in that car crash. I used to be proud of my strength, but what is that now? I now see and acknowledge the hand of God in my doom. I experienced remorse, and that finally led to repentance. My one purpose in life now is to help disabled people as much as I can in my remaining years.

Peter had become a happier person, in spite of his disabilities, and he had acquired a new serenity and purpose in life which had completely obliterated his old philosophy.

A Patient's Letter

Most patients express their feelings in dialogue with their gynaecologist and this book contains a number of case histories which play out their stories. Some, however, preferred to write down their inmost, emotional sentiments. I received more than twenty such letters and submit one that is representive. It has been printed in its entirety:

The letter

I am writing regarding an issue of the utmost importance to us all: that of human life and its value.

I have been one of the many to have made the fatal mistake of choosing abortion as an alternative to an untimely pregnancy.

I am in two minds whilst writing this as I do not wish to cause hurt to those who have chosen abortion as I did, but rather to help those who may be faced with such a decision, either now or in the future. I feel it is about time that the consequences of this decision for many women has to be aired. This is the other side of the coin which has been 'brushed under the carpet'.

I feel it my duty to fellow women and their unborn to speak up and make others realize that to abort an unborn child can, and does, have disastrous results.

By dealing with the pregnancy this way it can be simply removing one problem to replace it with one far worse.

Pregnancy was God's idea. Abortion Man's. Woman was not made to deal with the consequences of abortion because it is a totally unnatural concept.

There are many women living in silent anguish in this society today after a very painful realization of what they have done to their own unborn. It must be shared with those who may fall prey to the same trap in the future.

I'm sure that if those, whose own personal experiences taught them such a hard lesson, would all come forward many a woman would review her own decision which is often hasty and uninformed. Sadly there are too many doctors in our society who do not do their jobs properly, for if they considered their first and foremost oaths as doctors, that of preserving human life to the best of their ability, they would all be counselling women very strongly to carry on the pregnancy.

Most would realize their reasons were hysterical and petty and would choose to keep the child and be far better off doing so, even if they hadn't thought so at the time; and adoption is still a far better alternative to the unborn than death, for both mother and child can walk in the knowledge that she cared enough to come to terms with adoption, if necessary. The adoptive parents, who desperately want a child, would be thrilled that the child's right to life was respected. Abortion is like trying to pretend a pregnancy never happened. But what of the woman left? She knows it happened, and that fact is merely balancing in the subconscious, and its repercussions will manifest themselves psychologically in the majority of women to greater and lesser degrees.

So many have become so blasé about abortion that I feel contraception and fear of pregnancy are treated so lightly because we have allowed our attitudes to become so degraded as to irresponsibly conceive human life, and just as irresponsibly to dispose of it, with barely an afterthought for that unique precious little individual whose right to live is as valid as yours or mine.

What has become of human beings that we are destroying our

own children and at the same time shout 'Save the whales, and save the Seals'? Let's face the truth of this rampant evil called ABORTION, and stamp out abortion first.

Save the human babies! Everyone supporting preservation of other forms of life are hypocrites unless they are supporting first and foremost the preservation of fellow man.

I am so angry at my own horrible selfishness, yet angry at a society whose evil values affected my thinking.

I see abortion now as the subtle evil it really is and, when one realizes this, it is a big pill to swallow for a human being who would normally never even be able to comprehend violence or the harming of others, and most women who have abortions are 'normal' people being brainwashed into accepting this abomination because society is offering women this alternative, without legal repercussions and, disgustingly, it has become so acceptable.

A woman will close her mind off to what she is really doing to her own child.

The same woman would fret for weeks if the family cat were run over. Subtle hypocrisy!!

It all comes back to a sick naïve destructive society where abortion is far too easily obtainable.

Radical Restrictions should be imposed for the sake of all concerned.

Abortion is a dirty word and should be treated as such. It is common knowledge that abortion is a big money spinner; this is particularly sickening.

My concern is for all these naïve sheep being wheeled into operating theatres, foolishly allowing their own young to be destroyed and, unwittingly, destroying a part of themselves in the process.

And the young people growing up today believing abortion is not such a bad thing because even many of their parents are accepting the outright murder of these little people being forcibly removed from their mothers' wombs. How many will, when the penny drops, regret, beyond words, this thing they have done? How resentful they will feel towards their elders for making this horrible thing available to them.

To anybody who supports abortion I would say, "I would take a long, hard look at how Evil is in control of your thinking. If you still prefer to condone abortion one day you will wake up to the truth." But how many more lives will these people be indirectly or directly involved in destroying before they do?

I say to these people, "You were fortunate that you were born in a time when abortion was not so prevalent or acceptable, or you may not be here today!"

What audacity have any of us to treat other human lives with less respect than we treat our own, regardless of what stage of development this life is at! If we all realized this, abortion would be rare indeed. And so it should be.

The sadness is that when women are faced with this decision they feel snowed under with all sorts of 'valid' reasons why they should terminate a pregnancy. It seems the easiest and best thing to do at the time.

They allow themselves to be pressured by husbands or boyfriends, so in they go..... not allowing themselves time to think of their child. And it is especially unfortunate when they do not come into contact with someone that supports right to life, because they cannot make a balanced decision.

I urge anyone who believes that abortion is wrong to speak up loudly and clearly to anyone they meet who is considering termination.

Your voice may save a life. These children are at the mercy of whoever is involved or aware of their possible fate. They cannot talk for themselves; someone has to be spokesperson for them.

I think you have gathered I have a full realization of the enormity of my mistake, hideous and irreversible. It is rather like being in a state of shock. A wiser person I am, but life is a painful place for me. Now I can be at peace in the knowledge that God has forgiven me for that tragic wrong decision, but prevention would have been far better than cure.

I could spend every waking moment for the rest of my life warning people that abortion can be the biggest mistake of their lives.

It is right and beautiful to allow our children to live in our tummies until it is time for them to be born. These defenceless little people are our own flesh and blood.

A PREGNANCY IS A REAL PERSON.

A Doctor's Letter

One obviously had many thousands of letters from General Practitioners during one's professional career referring patients for assessment and treatment, but it must also be remembered that, from time to time, Gynaecological colleagues also referred patients for treatment if one happened to have special expertise in certain operative procedures. I therefore include one sent from a London Teaching Hospital as an example. The patient's and the referring colleague's names have been changed to avoid identification, and the Hospital, likewise, is not identified:

Dear Dr Chapman

Re: Charlotte ********

This lady was seen in January of 1985 under the care of Professor ********. I understand in 1973 or 4 she had a hysterotomy at 8 weeks gestation for an unknown reason. In 1977 she had a spontaneous rupture of the uterus at 35 – 36 weeks gestation; the baby living for two days. The following year she ruptured her uterus again at 30 weeks gestation; the baby living for one hour. Both these disasters occurred at ***** ****'s Hospital, **********, She was admitted in March 1985 for hysteroscopy, laparoscopy and laparotomy. At hysteroscopy intrauterine synechiae were found; there was noted to be a pale 1 cm wide anterior scar. Because of dense adhesions a laparotomy was performed through a lower transverse incision. The uterus was noted to be densely adherent to the anterior abdominal wall at the fundus, and to the bladder. Both tubes and ovaries were reported as being normal. There were dense adhesions to the bowel, omentum, and anterior abdominal wall and uterus. The fundus of the uterus was dissected free, but attempt of separation of the bladder from the uterine scar was abandoned because of risk to the bladder. In the April of 1985, I understand, the husband was going to have a vasectomy. She was last seen in March 1987 for an intrauterine contraceptive device check. A multiload 250 was in her uterus.

In summary, this lady has had a hysterotomy followed by spontaneous ruptures of the uterus, associated with neonatal deaths. Intra-abdominally there are numerous adhesions, and the anterior part of the uterus is not visible due to adhesions to the anterior abdominal wall and bladder.

Wishing you the very best of luck!

Yours sincerely,

Nick *********

Senior Registrar

It is perhaps desirable to explain what a hysterotomy is, for it is not an operation that is commonly employed these days. It is, essentially, a type of Caesarean section employed to deliver a foetus as an alternative to vaginal termination of pregnancy. Employed in the past quite commonly for late terminations, and employed by the gynaecologist to deliver the twins described in, "The Doctors' Lounge", it has largely been superseded by other methods. The lower part of the uterus in the first and second trimesters of pregnancy has not become thin. The consequence is that very thick uterine muscle has to be divided to reach the foetus. As a result, in future pregnancies the uterine scar is prone to rupture. Why the patient described in the letter had a hysterotomy performed at eight weeks gestation is not known. Presumably, however, the uterus was perforated during an attempted vaginal termination and the gynaecologist thought it wisest to complete the termination by the abdominal route. The other surgical operations mentioned in the letter have been adequately described in previous sections of the book.

The letter is included to demonstrate some further quite serious complications that can occur in women who have been promised a 'simple termination'.

A Russian Story

I am immensely grateful to my dear friend and colleague, Professor Marius S. Plouzhnikov, for allowing me to include the following true story that he has written:

Polina

by M S Pluzhnikov

In everlasting memory
of my aunt Alexandra.

"Envy is the enemy
of happiness".
From "Conversations" by
Epictetus.

It was 1944. I had finished technical college just before the war and was assigned to the tiny village of Rakhya on the road to Ladoga as assistant to an accountant for a peatery. I was stuck there for a long time.

Our manager was called Syerov – a taciturn, stout old man, breathless from a weak heart. The people working there were all women; they were exhausted and always dirty. They wore quilted jackets and heavy tarpaulin boots. Nobody's life was private; each knew everybody and everybody knew each, his or her sorrows and misfortunes. They were waiting for the end of the war and thought of nothing else.

The only bright patch in this joyless pattern of life was Polina. She reminded everybody of their best years and I suspect that many of the women went to the Manager's room with the sole purpose of catching a glimpse of her and reminding themselves of how they had been in that pre-war time, now lost to them for ever. They very much loved her for her kindness and humanity and, it would seem, drew some strength from her.

It happened that I took some registers to Syerov for signature. Polina was sitting at her secretarial desk and talking on the phone. She was older than I by about five years and slightly shorter. Her slender, graceful figure was clad in a modest brown suit and impeccably snow-white blouse with a turn-down collar. Finishing her telephone conversation she turned her pretty face to me and looking directly at me, her big brown eyes shining with warmth and gentleness, she smiled.

Quite spontaneously we started to talk. She asked me about myself and without thinking I chatted to her about the sort of nonsense typical of a young girl of my age. I told her I read nothing as we did not have a library, and she gladly invited me to her home to choose something interesting.

Polina had a large, bright room of 14 metres, with two windows. Clean curtains, a white cloth and well arranged old furniture created an atmosphere of comfort and human warmth.

I had hardly entered, than the door opened behind me and Polina's fat neighbour Dusya, the woman employed to check our daily work quotas, barged into the room without knocking.

"It crossed my mind the girls had thought something up and that I'd drop in" – she spoke noisily, direct from the threshold – "I was thinking that if you've got such a guest, it would be nice to have some tea, eh?"

Polina remembered that she hadn't offered me anything to eat or drink but Dusya, not pausing for a moment, and as though it were perfectly normal, continued: "And what's tea! Some cold, salted potatoes would be nice too!"

Embarrassed, Polina fetched some cold unpeeled boiled potatoes, placing them ceremoniously on little plates. With her nimble finger nails, Dusya began to tear one from its skin and thrust it into her mouth, dipping it in salt. Without chewing it properly, her mouth still full, she did not leave, and laughing, she suddenly declared:

"Come on then. You should offer your guests some of the tinned food your boy friend brought. There it is. I can see the edge of the tin sticking out from behind the newspaper."

Polina flushed crimson, her fingers began to tremble and she fetched the tin of fish in tomato sauce.

"That's nice," said Dusya approvingly, but at that point I began to protest strongly that there could be no question of opening the tin. This clearly disappointed Dusya.

She devoured three potatoes, finished her loud chewing and sighed. Folding her hands on her stomach, she said:

"I envy you, Pol'ka. You're lucky. What a room you have. Mine is so poky, there's no room in it for someone of my build to sit or stand. And what a man you've got yourself – so handsome. Some people have everything and others nothing – like me, for instance. So much good gone to waste," and she laughed sensuously, supporting her swaying, powerful breasts with her hands.

Polina's face darkened and, restraining herself, she looked reproachfully at Dusya. Dusya realised that she had said too much, jumped up from the stool and blurted anxiously:

"But that was only an example, Polyechka – nothing more. Eat, eat girls and I'll be off. I've lots to do," and she made her way to the door, her boots thudding.

All our women disliked Dusya, but feared her. Whether or not we satisfied our work quotas was decided by her and her colleague Mashka Voronova, and quotas were a rule of war time. It didn't take long for people to get summoned to the tribunal.

Mashka was uncouth but fair, but Dus'ka had no scruples about extorting rations and everybody could see her grow as fat as a pig. I knew that behind her back she was called a "branded witch" because of her pockmarks.

I would have protested at Dus'ka's ill mannered intrusion and her rude comments, but Polina put her hand on my shoulder and said calmly:

"Don't, Ninochka. I know what you want to say. Dusya is a simple woman. Simple women are finding things particularly difficult just now. Don't let's judge anybody. You see, we must be above that sort of thing. Let's talk about books instead," and she led me to her cherished bookshelf.

When Nina left, Polyenka took out her hairpins and began sadly to examine the little wrinkles on her face. Then she took a photograph from the top drawer of the chest and looked at Sasha. The photograph showed him still in his naval training uniform and peakless cap. He gazed at her frankly and she vividly recalled everything that had happened. After the graduation ball at the Herzen Institute the whole group went to the Neva. It was a warm white night. When they reached the Bronze Horseman, somebody suggested: "Girls, let's go to the dance at the Marble Palace. They'll be in full swing there." No-one agreed at once, arguing that it was late and a long way to go.

Just then a cheerful group of fresh naval graduates appeared, all wearing new officers' uniforms. They joined hands and laughingly encircled the girls in a tight ring, not allowing any of them to pass through. "We'll go with you, girls", they cried. A tall, dark young man whose uniform fitted him like a glove came up to Polyenka and saluted her. Not expecting this, she took his arm and they slowly moved through the night time city. They were both shy to begin with, but soon got into conversation. They reminisced about their teachers, their exams and various amusing incidents, each recalling friends and relatives. Sasha told her he was due to join a submarine and Polyenka mentioned that she had been assigned to a school in Rakhya. They decided not to go to the Marble Palace, and he took Polyechka home. Twice he attempted a clumsy kiss, but she deftly avoided him, laughing. They lingered by the front door and she herself suddenly planted a farewell kiss on his cheek. Dumbfounded, he stood for a long time, rubbing his cheek.

It turned out that the position at the school was already taken, but she got a job as secretary to Syerov. The war was already well under way and there wasn't much choice.

She never stopped thinking about Sasha. In November 1942 she called at the school for the umpteenth time and was at last given a long lost triangular envelope showing a field post office number. The letter had been heavily daubed by the censor, but the gist of it was intact.

"Dear Polyenka," wrote Sasha and quoting Simonov, "I shall return in defiance of death, but you must be very patient. All my love, Sasha."

And she waited throughout the war. She received no reply to her long, detailed letter. Then, for some reason, she unravelled her mother's cardigan and knitted him socks, although it was probably not at all cold in the submarine, and she sent him the small parcel not even knowing whether this sign of attention would reach him.

In 1944, churning the muddy soil with its strong tyres, a Studebaker ground to a halt beneath the windows of her room. It had barely stopped when out jumped a tall, handsome lieutenant. He instantly rushed up to her door, as though sensing where she must be. Polyenka hardly had time to draw in her breath before he flew into the room, slinging down his precious gifts at random, lifted her into his arms as though she were a feather, and whirled her round and round, kissing her. The Studebaker did not wait for him, and Sasha spent the night with her. They had seven such meetings before he said he would be going to sea for a long time.

Polyenka lay on the bed and remembered that when they had awoken in the morning for the last time, Sasha had whispered, stroking her head gently:

"My darling little reed. There isn't and never will be anybody in the whole world dearer to me than you".

About ten days after I visited Polina, Dusya came into the accounts office, cautiously shutting the door behind her. "Hallo, everybody," she said politely, looking principally at our stern chief accountant. "I am wondering if I could have an advance. I'm being sent on a business trip to St Petersburg." The chief accountant looked up from her papers, looked at Dusya coldly and snapped:

"You will have the standard 24-hour travel allowance if you show me documentary evidence that you are being sent on business to St Petersburg." Dusya shifted from one leg to the other and spun right round without saying goodbye. As she slammed the door behind her, she could be heard loudly blurting in the corridor: "Silly old bag. Get stuffed."

Work helped to occupy Polina, but for some reason, alarming thoughts about Sasha crowded in on her that day, and she was filled by vague foreboding. It was a terribly difficult day. She and Syerov were worn out and she only just managed to get home. She felt sick. Nobody knew she was three months pregnant.

The door of Polina's room creaked and in her usual simple way, but this time a little tipsy, Dusya barged in.

"Polya, Polya – listen," she warbled. "What shall I tell you?" and leaning against the wall in her quilted coat, "Miracles! Do you know whom I saw in St Petersburg? You won't guess! Your Sasha!"

Polyenka sensed something bad, and started to feel giddy. As she was standing, she feverishly grasped the back of a chair in order to keep her balance.

"Hallo," he says, and there he is with a queen on his arm, a blond girl. By the Holy Cross! "This is my lawful wife," he says. "Allow me to introduce Valentina Ivanovna." And I says, "What do you mean?" and he laughs and he says: "That's how it is."

"Men! They're all heathen dogs. If only they …………"

But Polyenka no longer heard Dusya. Her pale lips stirred without a sound.

"So now you're a field wife. They're all dogs. Spit on them and have done with them. That's all there is to say," added Dusya decisively.

Half conscious, Polyenka continued to whisper something. Images of the past flashed through her mind and the word "child" hummed in her ears like a steeple bell.

Dusya listened and understood.

That's nothing," she said. "I'll go straight away to ………." and she vanished through the door,

Polyenka didn't see Dusya leave, but continued standing motionless on her weakening legs, gripping the chair. Then she quietly sank down onto the floor.

When she came to, she felt that something irreversible had happened and, at once recollecting, she began to groan from the excruciating pain. Gradually her thoughts resumed their former clarity. She simply could not believe that her Sasha, so gentle and so dear to her, was capable of this.

"It's not true. It can't have happened. There must be some mistake. Something doesn't fit," she thought. But suddenly she felt shattered by the full force of the insult inflicted upon her and her life lost its sense. Something was torn asunder within her and, weeping dully, she fell onto the bed.

"What are you howling for, you simple soul?" asked Dusya, sympathising with her from somewhere above her. "Is he worth it, the traitor? By the Holy Cross, I've been saying to Semyonovna that Sashka is a traitor."

Polyenka half rose and saw the smiling old woman seated above her.

"My daughter," she intoned, "Don't grieve. There have been

so many like you in my time. And you'll forget everything, darling. Women are so tenacious of life. It'll all pass, darling. O God, it'll pass. I'll wash my hands with soap and I'll see to everything. Semyonovna has helped many, my darling, in her time. But give me two tins of fish. My grandson is starving."

By morning Polya was unrecognisable. Her darkened face was flushed crimson. Syerov looked in on her, casually the first time, but then more attentively, and asked anxiously: "Polina Vasilyevna, what's the matter? You must go to the doctor at once, I beseech you."

Utterly confused, she managed to get home. Every step was painful. Once there, she immediately lay down. She began to dream, and then lost consciousness completely.

Towards evening Dus'ka told the doctor's assistant everything.

"Such people should be brought to justice," he said, but mentioned no names. And he went to Polyenka. He wrapped her in a blanket – she had grown very thin in the last 24 hours – and carried her easily to his car. For an instant she regained consciousness, and it seemed to her that her beloved Sasha was holding her in his arms and rocking her like a small child, tenderly kissing her, and she could hear her mother saying:

"My little daughter. We'll go to the school fête and you'll put on your white dress which I bought for you for the New Year."
But the next morning, she was no more.

The village was shaken by Polenka's death. For a time people forgot their troubles and were only aware of their common tragic loss.

The day after Polyenka's funeral Dus'ka called on Syerov with a request that he give her Polina's room as she was his best worker and a close friend of Polina and, without a word, Syerov wrote boldly in the top left hand corner of the paper: "Request granted."

It was a wonderful spring with flowering grasses and the scent of fresh leaves.

A tall, broad shouldered, happy faced captain of the 3rd Rank alighted from a passing car and went to the house where Polyenka had once lived. He opened the door of her room and saw the same furniture there, but the whole scene looked uncomfortable and untidy. On the wall hung a tiny photograph in a black frame and at the table sat Dusya eating potatoes and onions.

He stopped at the door in astonishment and looked at her, puzzled.

"Why don't you greet me, Sasha?" asked Dus'ka belching. "Don't you recognise me?"

"Hallo, Dusya," he said politely. "And where is my Polenka?" Where is she? She's dead. That's where she is – in the graveyard. She died from an abortion."

He swayed, and his rucksack crashed to the floor. As white as a sheet, Sasha seized the door post and went limp, like an old man.

News of his arrival spread like lighting through the village. The women came running from their houses, putting on their scarves. The two of them came out, Dus'ka in the lead, and he behind her. We saw everything and followed them to the cemetery, keeping a distance from them. Suddenly we heard a heart-rending shriek and sobbing. We ran immediately to the cemetery.

It was terrible to see how that strong man and sailor suffered. In his naval uniform he lay with his arms around the grave, his whole body convulsing. His fingers dug deep into the soil and he frenziedly called her to him, repeating:

"Come back, come back. I am here. I am here with you!!!!"

One of the women gave a pitiful howl, lamenting. He leaped to his feet, not understanding anything, and stared at us.

Then Mashka Voronova couldn't stand it any more, stepped out in front and, pointing her finger at Dus'ka, shrieked:

"It was she, she – the branded whore!" and breaking into sobs all the time, she told him everything.

He raised his hands to the sky. He looked at us and then at Dus'ka. He looked her in the eye and in anguish he repeated: "Why? Why? Why? I have nobody – no relations. I am an orphan!"

The whole village gathered at the office. The women wept and threatened Dus'ka. Syerov came out, Dus'ka following him, hiding behind him.

"I have put right what I could," he said breathlessly, his eyes downcast. "She will no longer have ………….." and he paused for a moment, and then added paternally "………….. Polyenka's room."

There was a noisy response. Someone shouted from the crowd,

"She won't live with us any more, the vile creature."

All my life I have remembered my Polyenka and the story of her and Sasha's tragic love. I used to ponder the question – and I ponder it even more now in my declining years, as I review past and present, the question which forever plagues me and leaves me no peace of mind:

"O God, why is there so much evil in the world?"

Warsaw, 17 March 1994

152

Why do Women have Abortions?

Abortion law reform was introduced, in most Western countries at least, in order to save those desperate women who might otherwise end up as casualties in the hands of the back street abortionists. But what of those women, and I have seen quite a number, who though they have no medical or social condition which might merit termination of pregnancy, nevertheless, request it because, "pregnancy, at the moment, is not convenient", although they frequently add that they would like to get pregnant in a few months time?

Can it be that certain physiological changes, which occur in women's bodies throughout the reproductive phase of their lives, are responsible for this rejection? I do not know the answer, but I think it appropriate to end this monograph by saying something about female and pregnancy hormones, and physiological and psychological changes which occur in pregnancy, and also the immunological capability of the embryo, in order to educate, but more importantly, in the hope that some scientist might be encouraged to investigate this important subject.

It is a great mystery that has puzzled me for years. On the one hand one has the mother who will sacrifice everything, even life itself, for her unborn baby or her child, and on the other there is the mother-to-be who demands that her unborn child is taken away . How can one explain these two irreconcilable features of motherhood? One rarely sees it in the animal kingdom. Why is it that man, who all consider to be the head of the animal kingdom, even if not all accept that man is created in the image of God, falls so far short of the lesser beasts in this respect?

No other love is so tender and true as the love of a mother for her child. It has inspired some of the world's most sublime art, music and poetry, and it illuminates much of my patients' medical records:

> Womanliness means only motherhood;
> All love begins and ends there, — rooms enough,
> But, having run the circle, rests at home.
> > R. Browning

Charles Churchill, too, writing a polemical poem in 1764 against the evils of the day, on the other hand, described in graphic detail the morality and spirituality of women:

> Woman, the pride and happiness of Man,
> Without whose soft endearments Nature's plan
> Had been a blank, and Life not worth a thought;
> Woman, by all the Loves and Graces taught,
> With softest arts, and sure, tho' hidden skill,
> To humanize, and mould us to her will;
> Woman, with more than common grace form'd here,
> With the persuasive language of a tear
> To melt the rugged temper of our Isle,
> Or win us to her purpose with a smile;
> Woman, by fate the quickest spur decreed,
> The fairest, best reward of ev'ry deed
> Which bears the stamp of honour

Even the infertile woman will undertake the most drastic regimen in the attempt to achieve a pregnancy. On the other hand, there are those women who reject their pregnancies and demand termination; and this too features in my records. How can these things be reconciled?

Can it be, I wondered, if some of these irreconcilable female inconsistencies are brought about by the fluctuating hormone levels that afflict the woman throughout adolescence, pregnancy, the monthly cycle and the menopause? We are all familiar with the changes in mood and behaviour of the teenaged girl, morning sickness that distresses so many of those in early pregnancy, postnatal depression, which has led some women to harm or abandon their babies, the premenstrual syndrome, which in extreme cases has resulted in murder, and the misery which some women experience during the long, drawn-out menopause. It is therefore incumbent on me to spend a little time in discussing the female hormones which can so distress the female of our species.

Hormones are chemically diverse substances that are released into the bloodstream in response to some stimulus and which activate cells and thereby regulate many processes throughout the body. They serve many important functions in our lives. Not only are hormones responsible for psychological and emotional changes, but they obviously cause physical changes, which are in fact their main action. There are many hormones in the body that cause all kinds of effects to regulate normal bodily function, but here we are only concerned with the female reproductive hormones.

Female Hormones:

In women there are many specialized female hormones that affect them from the beginning of life right into old age, so it is important to learn as much as possible about them.

As we grow up from childhood and begin to develop, hormones, previously held dormant, begin to be released and cause many changes in physical appearance. They also bring about many internal differences as well. Female hormones are responsible for all the specialized development that a girl goes through in becoming a woman. The process usually takes around four years and during this time varying hormone levels can be difficult to adapt to. When the process begins, the hypothalamus, which is an integral part of the brain, starts to release hormones that will in turn trigger another endocrine gland, the pituitary gland. The pituitary gland is a tiny, pea-sized structure that hangs down on a stalk from the hypothalamus at the base of the brain. In addition to other hormones, it releases the luteinising hormone (LH) and the follicle stimulating hormone (FSH). They act on the ovaries, which are then stimulated to create their own female hormones.

Female hormones are also necessary to regulate a woman's menstrual cycle, are required to maintain pregnancy and are needed for childbirth. The main hormones produced by the ovaries are progesterone and oestrogen. These, together with LH and FSH, have a large role to play in a women's natural cycle.

Hormones drastically change when a woman becomes pregnant. Oestrogen and Progesterone levels remain high in the body during this time. Other hormones also play their part and each hormone involved in pregnancy serves a vital role in this complex cycle.

After a pregnancy has been completed hormone levels yet again take another remarkable change and revert back to normal levels. This can be difficult for some women to adapt to and there are a number of negative symptoms that are believed to be caused by the many hormonal changes occurring in the body at this time. Female hormones and their effect on emotional and psychological behaviour are still not fully understood.

Women undergo another change in hormone levels at around the age of 45 to 50 years. At this point the ovaries become unable to produce normal amounts of female hormones. This is known as the menopause. When the process begins there may be irregularities in the menstrual cycle until, finally, it ceases altogether. This can have a negative effect on many aspects of health since oestrogen serves many functions, including protecting the heart and bones. There are also various other negative side effects caused by the menopause such as hot flushes and bone loss. There are, however, a number of ways to treat such side effects, including hormone replacement therapy. Hormone replacement therapy may even be able to protect against osteoporosis and heart disease. However, this therapy requires a balance that should be further discussed with whoever prescribes HRT for you.

Thus, from the very beginning of life, female hormones have a great effect on a woman's life. They shape appearances, make having children possible and are responsible for many important experiences of women. Knowing all you can about these important aspects of your body is important for keeping you healthy.

Prgnancy hormones:

Human Chorionic Gonadotropin (hCG), which is a hormone produced by the placenta to maintain the corpus luteum (the change that occurs in the ovarian follicle after ovulation has occurred) during pregnancy, stimulates the production of oestrogen and progesterone within the ovary. It is released very early in pregnancy and is not present at any other time. This is the hormone which pregnancy tests look for. Production of this hormone diminishes once the placenta is mature enough to take over oestrogen and progesterone production.

Oestrogen causes the breast tenderness and enlargement that are typical of early pregnancy. It is produced throughout pregnancy, and helps to regulate levels of progesterone and to prepare the womb for the baby and the breasts for feeding.

Progesterone prevents the womb from spontaneously aborting the foetus by building up the lining so that it can support the placenta, and by preventing the natural movement and contractions of the womb. This is the hormone that is responsible for the loss of interest in sex during pregnancy.

Prolactin is produced by the pituitary gland. It is responsible for the increase in cells which produce milk within the breasts. Progesterone and oestrogen actually prevent milk from being produced. Immediately after birth, the levels of these hormones drop dramatically, allowing prolactin to stimulate the initial production of milk. Suckling also controls milk production. Prolactin also helps to prevent a nursing mother from falling pregnant, but cannot be relied upon as the only form of contraception.

Relaxin is found early in pregnancy and is responsible for helping to limit the activity of the womb and to soften the cervix in preparation for delivery.

Oxytocin seems to be involved in reproductive behaviour in both men and women, and apparently triggers 'caring' behaviour. It is also the hormone that allows contractions of the womb during pregnancy and labour. Contractions felt during breast feeding are also due to oxytocin. It can also be used to induce labour.

Prostaglandins are tissue hormones that seem to play a role in getting labour started. Synthetic prostaglandins are also used to induce labour in a pregnancy which has gone past its 40th week.

Psychological Changes in Pregnancy:

While a woman experiences radical physiological changes during the months before birth, every mother-to-be also undergoes profound psychological changes. Becoming a mother for the first time is a major milestone in any woman's development. It is a time when a woman revisits her own childhood and her early relationship with her mother as she considers whom she will emulate.

Pregnancy and new motherhood take a woman home. Home to her first intimate relationship. Home to her parents' marriage. Home to her earliest feelings of vulnerability and dependency. Each of us was once a vulnerable baby and small child, and we carry those earliest feelings inscribed in our brains.

What causes psychological changes during pregnancy?
The main reason for psychological changes that occur during pregnancy is because of the physiological changes that may be seen or are often unseen. The changing bodily shape, the increas-

158

ing body weight, and the changed levels of hormones are the main causes that are responsible for creating the unique mental state in pregnancy.

One of the conditions which is common and is peculiar to pregnancy is morning sickness. Nausea and vomiting during pregnancy, commonly known as "morning sickness," affects approximately 80% of pregnant women. Most of the time it is mild and settles by the twelfth week of pregnancy. On rare occasions it is very severe and is called hyperemesis gravidarum.

Hyperemesis gravidarum, a severe form of nausea and vomiting, affects one in 200 pregnant women. Although the definition of this condition has not been standardized, accepted clinical features include persistent vomiting, dehydration, ketosis (ketone bodies collecting in the blood in large amounts due to the vomiting, starvaton and electrolyte inbalance), electrolyte disturbances, and weight loss of more than 5% of body weight. If untreated it can endanger life. The British literary author, Charlotte Brontë, is said to have died from hyperemesis gravidarum. Today's safer therapeutic treatments and progressive medical thinking have helped those suffering from nausea and vomiting of pregnancy. The cause of the sickness is unknown.

What hypotheses have been propounded to explain hyperemesis gravidarum?

* Hormonal: Excess of chorionic gonadotrophin, proved by the frequency of vomiting at the peak level of hCG and also by its increased association with hydatidiform mole (a kind of malignancy) or multiple pregnancy when the hCG titre is very much raised.

* Psychogenic: It probably aggravates the nausea once it begins.

* Dietetic: deficiency: Probably due to low carbohydrate reserve, since it happens after a night without food. Deficiency of vitamin B6, vitamin B1 and proteins may be the effects rather than the cause.

* Allergic: May be related to some products secreted from

the ovum

*   Immunological basis.

*   Is the desire for termination also a type of sickness related to hormones?

One hundred years ago, on June 20th 1905, the English physiologist, Ernest Starling, brought the word 'hormone' into the public arena for the very first time. So many advances have been made in the realm of endocrinology since then, but we still have many unanswered questions in the realm of the physiology of pregnancy. I was privileged to work in Ruakura Animal Research Centre in New Zealand during the 1970s and had a chance to meet with Professor Sir Graham C. Liggins who was, even in those days, working on the physiology of parturition (childbirth). Nevertheless, it is obvious that we still need more research in reproductive physiology and endocrinology.

Those who are familiar with the need for life-long treatment with drugs to prevent a donated organ from being rejected by the recipient may well ask why it is that no similar aid is required by the developing foetus to prevent it from being rejected and expelled. It is important, therefore, that I now say a few words about the immunological problems facing the implanting embryo.

The Immunological Capacity of the Embryo:

One of the most amazing things associated with conception is the fact that the mother's body does not reject the growing foetus, in contra-distinction to what happens when a surgeon transplants a donated organ. In the latter case the graft has to battle with the host's immune system which strives to rid the body of the foreign invader. The cells that bear the major responsibility for carrying out the activities of the immune system are called lymphocytes. They are some of the white blood cells in the body and consist of the recipient's B lymphocytes that recognise antigens on the surface of the foreign cells as 'non-self' and manufacture antibodies against them. These antibodies then bind with the antigens and attempt their removal from the body. The other lymphocytes, that are processed in the thymus, are termed T lymphocytes. They also play an important role via cell-mediated immunity.

The patient who has received a donated organ thereafter requires lifelong treatment with an anti-rejection drug. Corticosteriods were originally used, but the most popular drug these days is the chemotherapeutic agent, cyclosporin, which is obtained from a poisonous Norwegian fungus. It has significant immunosuppressant properties which inhibit the action of the T lymphocytes that initiate the attack on the transplanted organ. Unfortunately the patient becomes more prone to infections because his or her immune system has been compromised.

If we now consider the implanting embryo we find that, amazingly, no rejection occurs. Many non-medical and non-scientific people imagine that the mother, by some means or other, succeeds in solving this problem, and this encourages many women to believe that it is 'their body' which they can do what they like with. In fact, the opposite is true. The embryo is the dominant partner in the relationship. When no larger than a grain of sand, he single-handedly solves the homograft problem (a homogrft is a tissue graft taken from a genetically nonidentical donor of the same species as the recipient).

Some six to eight days, commonly, after conception he sheds his capsule, and as the new surface is sticky, he implants wherever he happens to be; normally, of course, within the uterus. His first job is to prevent the menstrual shedding of his mother's endometrium. He does this by producing chorionic gonadotrophin which prolongs the life span of the corpus luteum in his mother's ovary. This, in turn, maintains the endometrium so that it can undergo a decidual reaction.

Soon after this the placenta, derived from the embryo and not from the mother it should be noted, takes over the production of the female sex hormones for the maintenance of the pregnancy, and the corpus luteum becomes redundant.

Finally, it should be pointed out that at the end of pregnancy he decides when he wishes to be born and initiates labour, that is, unless a doctor or midwife intervenes. The way that this was solved is so interesting that the readers are begged their indulgence while it is elaborated.

It is true that Hippocrates believed that the baby decided when he wished to be born, but this for centuries had been considered to be an old wife's tale. However, in 1933 Percy Malpas, a British obstetrician, noted that pregnancies were prolonged when the babies were anencephalic, i.e. in those in which part of their brains and skull bones were missing. Those observations suggested to some research scientists that the critical signals which started the birth process were possibly missing because they were lodged in that part of the brain that was absent in such anencephalic babies.

In the early 1960s reports emanated from the United States that two cows and one sheep that had unborn offspring with foetal abnormalities similar to human anencephalic foetuses, in which the pituitary endocrine gland and the hypothalamus were missing, also failed to go into labour.

Controlled experimental studies of the brains of foetal sheep were begun by Professor Sir Graham C. Liggins, an obstetrician in the National Womens' Hospital, Auckland, New Zealand, in the late 1960s, and he firmly established the fact that in sheep the foetus is the originator of the signal that initiates the birth process. He also discovered that the foetal pituitary and adrenal endocrine glands were the major means by which the birth process was begun.

He further confirmed that the same hormones produced by the foetus to start the birth process were also involved in maturing the foetal lungs so that they would be capable of breathing air after birth. This latter observation has enabled obstetricians to give steroids (normally manufactured by the adrenal gland) to mothers in impending premature labour, to accelerate lung maturity, and so enable such pre-term babies to survive.

This series of studies, designed to determine the critical factors that regulate the duration of pregnancy, is an excellent example of the value of basic scientific research, and the use of animal models to unlock the secrets of foetal development and to lead to better clinical care of the immature, pre-term baby.

We have not, as yet, discussed how the embryo solves the homograft problem. Firstly, the high concentration of progesterone produced by the placenta is known to kill the maternal lymphocytes, critical to the immune response. Secondly, placental cells have been shown to express an enzyme, indoleamine 2,3-dioxygenase, that locally disables the mother's immune system. Thirdly, it has recently been shown that a stress hormone, corticotrophin-releasing hormone (CRH), produced by the trophoblast, that will later form part of the placenta, induces the trophoblast to secrete a protein called Fas ligand, which is a transmembrane protein that belongs to the tumour necrosis factor. This protein fits into the Fas molecule on the surface of the T lymphocytes, like a key in a lock, and causes the T cells to enter an apoptotic stage that results in T cell suicide.

We have not said anything so far about the embryological development of the foetus. It is a vast subject which really falls outside the scope of this book. However, it might be worth mentioning that two weeks after the mother has missed her first period the baby is a quarter of an inch long, has a brain of human proportions, and has ears, eyes, mouth, liver, kidneys, and an umbilical cord with a heart pumping blood made by himself.

For thousands of years mankind had no personal experience of the development of the unborn child and might have been excused for believing that it could be dispensed with. However, during the last half century science has been unravelling its secrets, and now, with the development of 3D and 4D ultrasound, mothers themselves are able to see their unborn children at rest and at play. We know that the foetus can develop illnesses in utero, some being now amenable to treatment. The cracking of the genetic code in the 1960s has further extended our knowledge and has shown that every human being is unique and is different from every other human being. How tragic that, as all these secrets of the unborn child are being unravelled and scientists have proved that mankind is human from conception, the Law affords him no protection, and an increasing concerted effort is being made by much of mankind to consider him to be a non-person who can be destroyed as an alleged cure for all personal and social ills!

Abortion History in Brief

Infertility, which was recognised by the Ancients, was generally considered to be punishment of the god(s).The ancient Egyptians and the Hebrews, too, have at least recorded induced abortion, but moral issues in surviving records were not discussed.

The other source of information about abortion in ancient times is the Bible. It is one of the best historical accounts of ancient human civilization. Even if it is not taken for its religious purpose, the Bible accurately describes the culture of the Hebrew people. From the beginning of the Hebrew nation, unborn life was seen to be just as precious as life after birth.

Abortion, in some form, has existed in the human race for millennia. Ancient tribes would sometimes be forced to move quickly, and pregnant women could slow down the entire tribe. Abuse of the woman's abdomen, and later abuse through excessive horseback riding, could cause the baby to be born prematurely. This baby was then either killed or left to die. Unfortunately, the mother also frequently died during the birthing process. Today abortion is much safer for the mother, but just as deadly for the child.

The first recorded evidence of induced abortion is from a Chinese document which records abortions performed upon royal concubines in China between the years 515 and 500 BC.

According to Chinese folklore, the legendary Emperor Shennong prescribed the use of mercury to induce abortions nearly 5,000 years ago. If this causes a shiver in ones spine, it is also as unpleasant to know what is going on at the present time. Comprehensive new data show that traditional family patterns in China, combined with tough, population-control measures, have resulted in female infanticide on a grand scale — close on 800,000 baby girls were abandoned or killed in a single region alone between 1970 and 1980.

When we come to consider ancient Greek civilization we begin to see that there was, even at that early stage, disagreement as to whether abortion should be permitted or not. Aristotle allowed it to be used as a form of contraception, with the proviso that it should only be performed before the foetus had "developed sensation", presumably before 'quickening' (the first foetal movements felt by a pregnant woman) had been experienced; whereas the Pythagoreans opposed it as they believed that life began at conception. This conflict has persisted throughout the centuries, but with most Jewish, Christian and Muslim religious leaders opposing it. Hinduism, too, generally considers abortion to be bad 'karma'.

China began trying to control its massive population growth in 1970 and introduced a one-child-per-family policy in 1980 — an approach that ran into huge resistance and was relaxed after 1986. Statistics since 1990 show that China's male-female imbalance still persists.

In India there are less than 93 women for every 100 men in the population. The accepted reason for such a disparity is the practice of female infanticide, prompted by a dowry system which requires the family to pay out a great deal of money when a female child is married. For a poor family the birth of a girl child can signal extreme hardship and the beginning of financial ruin.

In old Russia termination of pregnancy was strictly forbidden, but after the Revolution in 1917 Russia was one of the first countries to legalise abortion in Europe and now has one of the highest rates of abortion in the world — three out of five pregnancies end in abortion.

In England, before the 19th Century, Common Law held that an abortion was only a misdemeanour if carried out before quickening, but in 1803 an Act was passed that made abortion a felony, both before and after quickening. In 1861 the Offences Against the Person Act revised penalties and made it an offence, not only for a woman to procure her own abortion, but also for anyone else who attempted to procure an abortion.

In the early 20the Century the Crimes Act sought to define when a child became a human being and it contained a section to protect obstetricians who might have to sacrifice a foetus to save the mother.

In 1938 Aleck Bourne, a prominent London gynaecologist, whom my husband, when a young doctor, later worked with, brought a test case after the rape of a 15-year-old girl by some soldiers. His defence was that the abortion had been carried out because continuing the pregnancy would make her a "physical or mental wreck". The judge's ruling was published in 1939 and led to a revised interpretation of the law.

In 1967 the Abortion Act was passed because of the disquiet felt at the number of deaths occurring as the result of 'back street abortionists'. It did not legalize abortions, but rather, provided a legal defence for those carrying them out. Essentially, it allowed abortion to be performed if continuance of a pregnancy involved greater physical or mental risk to a woman than having a termination of pregnancy. The patient's foreseeable future environment was also allowed to be taken into account, as was the likelihood that the child, if born, would be likely to suffer from serious physical or mental disabilities. The abortion needed to be agreed to by two doctors and carried out in a government approved hospital or clinic.

As with all permissive legislation it rapidly became abused. The numbers of women seeking abortion rose exponentially with many women using it as a form of contraception. Even Aleck Bourne became a persuasive critic because he realised that what the new law had been intended humanely to deal with in exceptional circumstances, soon became interpreted as allowing abortion on demand. He became a founder member of the Society for the Protection of the Unborn Child. In 2003 more than 192,000 abortions were performed in Great Britain and a further 9,100 on non-residents.

As in the case of Great Britain, abortion laws did not exist in the rest of Europe until the 19th Century. In 1869 Pope Pius IX declared that the soul entered the body at conception, and this led to restrictive legislation on abortion which still persists in much of South America and in some developing countries in Africa and Asia. In Muslim countries abortion is illegal unless the mother's life is in danger. However, in Europe between 1950 and 1985 most countries liberalized their abortion laws.

In Italy abortion is now legal on demand up to the 12the week of pregnancy, while in Spain and Portugal it was only legal up to the 12th week in cases of rape, foetal abnormality, or where there is danger to the mother's life or mental health. However, since 10th April 2007 the Portuguese parliament has widened the permissive nature of the law to bring it into line with most of its European neighbours.

In France, Germany and Denmark abortion is legal up to the 12th week of pregnancy, although in Germany it is compulsory for the mother to produce a certificate to the effect that she has consulted a counsellor.

Norway and Sweden allow abortion up to the 18th week of pregnancy, wheras in Switzerland it is illegal, unless the mother's life is ar risk. In Ireland it is also illegal, although it is interesting to note that in Northern Ireland there is no specific law either allowing or prohibiting abortion, in spite of the liberal law of the rest of the United Kingdom. In practice it appears to be rarely employed.

Poland allows abortion only for strictly medical reasons, while

Romania, on the other hand, which was the only country to prohibit abortion while under Communist rule, is now the most liberal, despite the fact that the limit is set at 12 weeks.

Were there laws against abortion in the early American colonies? The colonies inherited English Common Law, and largely operated under it until well into the 19th Century. English Common Law forbade abortion. Abortion prior to quickening was a misdemeanour. Abortion after quickening (foetal movments felt for the first time by the mother) was a felony. This bifid punishment, inherited from earlier ecclesiastic law, stemmed from earlier 'knowledge' regarding human reproduction. When did this change? In the early 1800s it was discovered that human life did not begin when the woman 'felt life', but, rather, at fertilization. As a direct result of this, the British Parliament, as we have seen, passed the "Offences Against the Persons Act", eliminating the bifid punishment and dropping the felony punishment back to fertilization. In 1967 Colorado and California legalized abortion and now most states, but not all, have followed this trend.

Methods of Abortion

T he reasons why it is necessary to write about the methods that are employed to perform terminations of pregnancy are twofold. Firstly it tells the woman who has chosen to have an abortion exactly what is involved and what risks she runs. Secondly, and more importantly, it says exactly what happens to the tiniest of humans who, without their consent, are subjected to this barbarous procedure. Is it not strange that there is public outcry when animals are maltreated, when animals are used for medical research, or when the huntsman gallops after a fox, but no voice is raised about the millions of human foetuses that are aborted each year?

Induced abortion can be defined as termination of pregnancy before the estimated date of delivery to ensure that the foetus does not survive. Some abortions occur naturally because a foetus does not develop normally or because the mother has an injury or disorder that prevents her from carrying the pregnancy to term (the time of expected delivery). This type of spontaneous abortion is commonly known as a miscarriage. Other abortions are induced, that is, intentionally brought on because a pregnancy is unwanted or because it presents a risk to a woman's health.

Different methods of induced abortion are used under different circumstances and at different stages of the development of the embryo or foetus. No method of abortion is 100% safe, and no method is 100% successful.

Induced abortion can be achieved by either medical or surgical intervention:

Medical Abortion:

Some of the earliest means of abortion included the ingestion of plants, herbs, or chemicals: The chemical methods that are used these days are as follows:

RU-486 or Misfepristone

Misfepristone, or Mifeprex, as it is called by the company that produces it, is an anti-progesterone that blocks the action of progesterone, which is one of the two hormones produced in the female body necessary to sustain a pregnancy.

This is the fastest growing abortion technique in the UK. This abortion pill blocks the effects of the hormone progesterone that is needed to maintain the lining of the uterus. This causes the lining to become detached along with the unborn child. It is usually used with another drug, a prostaglandin, which helps to dilate or open the cervix (the entrance to the womb) and expel the foetus.

The most common side effects that have been described are uterine cramping, bleeding, nausea and fatigue. The labelling for mifepristone emphasizes that cramping and bleeding are the primary side effects. Bleeding and spotting usually last for about nine to sixteen days. Heavy bleeding is possible, but rare. In about one in every 100 women the bleeding becomes heavy enough to require a surgical procedure to stop it.

The method of abortion consists of three tablets of the drug RU486 being taken together. Two days later a prostaglandin (see next page) pessary is inserted in the vagina. Within a few hours bleeding starts, and the embryo is lost with the blood. Bleeding continues for about 12 days, sometimes longer.

It has recently been reported that a woman became pregnant, much to her husband's displeasure, so he surreptitiously put a couple of RU-486 pills in her drink, without her being privy of the fact. She miscarried, and later became aware of her husband's dissimulation. She was incensed and her friends suggested that she should take him to court. If she does, what will he be charged with?

Prostaglandin

Prostaglandins are potent hormone-like substances that are produced in various mammalian tissues. They are derived from arachidonic acid, and mediate a wide range of physiological functions, such as control of blood pressure, contraction of smooth muscle, and modulation of inflammation

Medical induction is possible using prostaglandins. Either vaginal pessaries, or one of two forms of prostaglandin injection are available.

Adverse effects of prostaglandins include nausea, vomiting, diarrhoea, hyperthermia, facial flushing, vasovagal symptoms, bronchospasm, and decreased seizure threshold. In women with severe kidney or liver disorders, the activity of the drug may be decreased. If so the dose needs to be increased.

Its first approved use was for "the induction of mid-trimester abortion" (pregnancy has been divided up by the medical profession into approximately three periods of three months). The hormone produces a violent labour and delivery of whatever size baby the mother carries. If the baby is old enough to survive the trauma of labour, it may be born alive, but it is usually too small to survive. In one article, among the complications listed, was "live birth"!

Research undertaken at the Oxford Obstetrical and Gynaecological Units showed that there was an increased incidence of spontaneous abortion and placenta praevia (a placenta lying at the bottom of the uterus and overlying, or encroaching upon the cervix, or neck, of the uterus) after prostaglandin-induced abortion.

Other medical literature noted further complications. Thus experience with one patient undergoing second trimester abortion induced by prostaglandin F2alpha administration was described as developing serious hypokalemia (deficiency of potassium in the blood) in association with cardiac arrhythmia following intra-amniotic administration of the drug. Further observations on a group of normal subjects receiving prostaglandin injections for induction of abortion also showed a small but significant serum hypokalemia after treatment

Blood loss of 250 ml or more, pyrexia, pelvic infection, readmissions, and blood transfusions were all encountered from time to time. A further report on a patient showed hypokalemic periodic paralysis with thyrotoxicosis (hyperthyroidism), while a 31-year-old Hispanic woman underwent three prostaglandin inductions for a second-trimester abortion. Her management was complicated by hyperthermia, nausea, vomiting, and diarrhoea. She developed isolated proximal muscle paralysis and sensory loss on the first post-abortion day.

Methotrexate

Methotrexate is a chemotherapeutic drug that is given for treatment of many types of cancer, and it has all the possible side effects of such chemotherapeutic drugs.

This procedure is performed in the early first trimester. Methotrexate is injected and begins to attack the cells surrounding the embryo. The embryo is deprived of food and oxygen, and eventually dies. Several days later, misoprostol (see below) is injected to trigger the expulsion of the embryo. This expulsion may not occur for as long as eight weeks, and the woman may bleed heavily. The actual expulsion may occur at any moment and in any place. In about 4% of cases, expulsion does not occur and surgery is required.

Misoprostol

Misoprostol, an E1 prostaglandin analogue, has been approved only for the treatment of gastric ulcer.

Misoprostol (brand name: Cytotec) is a prostaglandin product that can be applied to the cervix to induce labour. It is also known as Prostaglandin E1, but it is not the same as the more common Prostaglandin E2 gel, Misoprostol is cheaper than Prostaglandin E2, and apparently the induction to delivery interval is reduced, but uterine hyperstimulation appears more likely to occur. The risk of uterine rupture is increased in those who have had previous Caesarean sections.

Finally one should realise that medical treatment of abortion is not always successful. If termination is not complete it could effect the baby and causes foetal abnormality, consequently surgical interference will be required.

Surgical Abortion:

Suction Aspiration (Vacuum Curettage)

The most common form of first trimester abortion is achieved by this method. The cervix is dilated, and a powerful vacuum tube with a sharp cutting edge is inserted. The suction rips apart the body of the baby, and sucks out blood, amniotic fluid, tissue, and body parts.

The most frequent post-abortion complications occur with this method. If any foetal or placental tissue is left behind in the uterus, infection can develop. Common side effects that most women experience include nausea, sweating, cramping and feeling faint. Less common complications include heavy or prolonged bleeding, passage of clots, and damage to the cervix or perforation of the uterus. Retention of some of the products of conception usually leads to infection, which causes fever, pain and abdominal tenderness, or the flare up of a previous sexually transmitted disease.

Dilatation and Curettage (D & C)

This is performed in the first trimester (up to the 12th week of pregnancy) and was commonly employed before suction aspiration had been introduced. The method involved dilatation of the cervix with graduated dilators and then the use of a large curette to dismember and break up the baby's body and thereafter their removal with ovum or sponge forceps.

This was a common method of abortion because it was used in early pregnancy and was not too dangerous for the woman. For this reason everyone rushed the pregnant women to have an abortion before she had had enough time to think. However, this had no scientific validity for the baby.

The side effects and possible complications are similar to those of suction curettage, although perforation of the uterus is slightly more common when this method is employed. If the uterus is perforated, the dilator or curette can also perforate the bladder, which will lead to peritonitis (infection of the peritoneum, or, in other words, the sac that covers and lines the abdominal contents) with consequent pain and the need for reparative surgery. Alternatively the intestines may be perforated, which will cause nausea, vomiting, abdominal pain, fever, blood in the stools, peritonitis and death, if not speedily treated by surgery. Should the latter arise the surgeon might have to resect a segment of bowel and also have to make a temporary or, very rarely, a permanent colostomy (formation of an alternative anus in the abdominal wall).

Between 2 and 3% of all patients undergoing abortion suffer perforation of their uterus. Most will remain undiagnosed unless bowel or bladder is also injured. Laparoscopy (telescopic inspection of the abdominal and pelvic contents through the abdominal wall) will usually be able to confirm the diagnosis. Risk of perforation is greater in the parous patient (one who has previously been pregnant) and in those whose termination has been performed under general anaesthesia. Uterine damage at the time of abortion, if not diagnosed, may give rise to further problems in later pregnancies.

Besides uterine perforations, significant cervical lacerations may also occur when the cervix is being dilated prior to evacuation of the uterine contents. Lesser tears can also lead to long-term reproductive damage resulting in cervical incompetence, premature delivery and complications of labour. Risks of these latter complications are greater in teenagers and in those who have undergone second trimester abortions.

Treatment of persistent bleeding following termination of pregnancy, usually by curettage, can also lead to problems, such as destruction of part or of all the endometrium (lining of the womb). This is called Asherman's Syndrome or uterine synechiae. It results in amenorrhoea (absence of periods) or hypomenorrhoea (scanty periods) and causes infertility. Intrauterine surgery with laser or other methods is required to treat this condition.

Salt Poisoning (Saline Injection)

This method has been used after the 16th week of pregnancy. A long needle is inserted through the mother's abdomen and uterine wall into the baby's amniotic sac. The baby swallows the deadly toxin and is poisoned. The mother delivers a dead or dying baby. This method can only be used after 16 weeks of pregnancy when enough fluid has accumulated in the amniotic sac surrounding the baby to enable the needle to be safely placed. Fifty to two hundred and fifty ml (as much as a cupful) of amniotic fluid is withdrawn and is replaced with a solution of concentrated salt. The chemical solution also causes painful burning and deterioration of the baby's skin. Usually, after about an hour, the child dies. The mother goes into labour about 33 to 35 hours after instillation of the salt solution and delivers a dead, burned, and shrivelled baby. About 97% of mothers deliver their dead babies within 72 hours.

Hypertonic saline (concentrated salt solution) may initiate a condition in the mother called "consumption coagulopathy" (uncontrolled blood clotting throughout the body) with severe haemorrhage as well as other serious side effects which affect the central nervous system. Seizures, coma, or death may also result from saline inadvertently injected into the woman's vascular system.

Urea Injection

Urea is a waste product of many living organisms, and is the major organic component of human urine. Urea injection is performed during the second or early third trimester. This is carried out in the same way as Salt Poisoning; however, it is not so strong, and therefore not as dangerous as Salt Poisoning.

Urea Injection increases the chance of a failed abortion, which usually results in surgery. Almost 2% of patients who have had

Urea Injections require to be hospitalized on account of side effects.

For both adults and teenagers up to 250ml are injected through the abdomen and the uterine wall into the amniotic sac after the same amount of fluid has been taken out. The injection may be repeated 48 hours after the first dose if it is needed.

Common side effects are nausea, vomiting, pain in the lower abdomen and weakness. Less common or rare complications include headache, diarrhoea, confusion, irregular heartbeat, unusual tiredness, muscle cramps or pain, numbness, tingling, weakness in hands or feet, and heaviness of the legs.

After the procedure is completed side effects may still occur that need medical attention, such as chills or shivering, fever, foul-smelling vaginal discharge, increase in bleeding from the uterus and pain in the lower abdomen.

Other side effects not listed here may also occur in some patients.

Hysterotomy or Caesarean Section

This is used mainly in the last three months of pregnancy, although in the past it was commonly employed in the second trimester. The uterus is entered by surgery through the anterior wall of the abdomen. The technique is similar to a Caesarean delivery, except that the umbilical cord is usually cut while the baby is still in the womb, thus cutting off his oxygen supply and causing him to suffocate. Sometimes the baby is removed alive and simply left in a corner to die of neglect or exposure.

Dilatation and Extraction (D & X)

After dilatation of the cervix ultrasound is used to guide the abortionist so that he can grab the baby's legs with forceps and pull them into the birth canal. They are then delivered, followed by the torso, arms and shoulders. The baby's head usually remains inside the uterus. Using blunt-tipped surgical scissors, the baby's skull is pierced after which a suction catheter is inserted to extract the 'skull contents', namely the brain. The skull then collapses and the dead baby is removed. Foetal brains and organs are sometimes used for foetal 'tissue' experimentation.

All abortions are traumatic, but late abortions particularly so. Whether carried out because of suspected foetal abnormality or not, they are extremely harrowing events, not only for the mother, but also for the attendant medical and nursing staff. Not only may the baby's cries be heard by all present if born alive, but those monitoring the event with 3D or 4D ultrasound, if intrauterine interference is being carried out, see the extreme anguish of the baby as they observe its violent movements and facial contortions and grimaces. For this reason, the Royal College of Obstetricians and Gynaecologists has issued guidelines, prepared by Scientific Authorities, for those carrying out late abortions: It states that in all late terminations the method chosen should ensure that the foetus is born dead. Intracardiac (within the heart) injection of potassium chloride is the recommended method, and the dose chosen should ensure that foetal asystole (cessation of heart beat) is achieved before prostaglandin induction. Continuous ultrasound monitoring is mandatory to confirm foetal, cardiac asystole, and, because the potassium chloride causes so much foetal distress, it is recommended that anaesthesia and muscle relaxant is instilled prior to the administration of the potassium chloride.

As an obstetrician I have two patients to consider: the mother and the child that she is carrying, and during my training I learnt, not only the skills required, but developed a love and compassion for the tiny baby for whom I was responsible. The baby also is given rights and the law permits him/her to sue me for negligence up to his/her age of twenty-one years. Babies are now surviving at 21 or 22 weeks and are given the protection of the law. What of those late abortions, often older than 21 weeks? The law is contradictory, and if young doctors witness the duplicity of their mentors and lose their compassion how can we expect them to provide the care that is expected?

Further Complications of Termination of Pregnancy

It is not generally recognised that abortion predisposes women to many forms of **cancer**. Nevertheless, this is the case that some research has shown. Women, who have had one abortion face an increased risk of developing cervical cancer, compared to non-aborted women, and those with two or more abortions an even greater risk. Similarly elevated risks for the development of ovarian and liver cancer also occur. Some studies have also shown that the risk of developing breast cancer almost doubles after one abortion and rises even further for two or more abortions. These increased cancer rates for post-aborted women are believed to be linked to the unnatural disruption of the hormone changes that accompany pregnancy, and to untreated cervical damage.

Abortion increases the risk of **placenta praevia** in later pregnancies by between seven and fifteen fold, while the abnormally low position of the placenta, caused usually in these cases by uterine damage, increases the risks of antenatal haemorrhage, foetal malformations and perinatal death.

Abortion significantly increases the risk of subsequent **ectopic pregnancy** which itself is life threatening.

Endometritis (Inflammation of the endometrium, or, in other words, inflammation of the lining of the uterus) has already been touched upon and is a post-abortion risk for all women, but especially for teenagers.

Pelvic Inflammatory Disease is a potentially life-threatening disease that can lead to an increased risk of reduced fertility and ectopic pregnancy. If patients have a chlamydial infection at the time of the abortion, 23% will develop pelvic inflammatory disease within one month. It is believed that a quarter of all patients seeking termination of pregnancy have a latent chlamydial infection. Finally, it has been shown that 5% of patients will develop pelvic inflammatory disease after undergoing a first trimester abortion even though they do not have a chlamydial infection at the time of the operation.

Asherman's Syndrome (intrautrine adhesions) is a condition in which the inner surfaces of the uterus stick together and ultimately form scar tissue which may be thick or thin, scanty or confluent. It may occur following uterine curettage made necessary because of retained pieces of placenta following child birth or spontaneous abortion, or it may simply occur after termination of pregnancy. It results in amenorrhoea (absent periods) or hypomenorrhoea (scanty periods). Treatment to be successful so that future pregnancies occur and do not end in spontaneous abortion requires that a laser surgeon should divide the adhesions through a hysteroscope. This book records the story of one patient who had developed Asherman's Syndrome.

Rhesus isoimmunization is another complication which can develop in rhesus negative women. Besides the ABO blood groups a rhesus facor is also present in most people. It is a protein that is present on th surface of the red cells. Should the woman who has the abortion be rhesus negative (not have the rhesus factor) while the father of her baby is rhesus positive, then her blood may not be compatible with that of her baby. Thus, when the abortion is performed the baby's blood may leak into hers and her immune system will start to produce antibodies against this rhesus positive blood. Should this occur, then the next time she is pregnant with a rhesus positive baby the antibodies will attack her new baby's blood. To avoid this possibility, all rhesus negative women having abortions should be give an injection of rhesus immune globulin. How often, one wonders, is this done in abortion clinics around the world?

This book has enumerated a number of patients who developed **psychological damage** as a result of their terminations. Research workers have found that 44% complained of nervous disorders, 36% experienced sleep disturbances, 31% regretted the decision that they had made, and 11% had been prescribed psychotropic medicine by their general practitioners. In a study from two Canadian Provinces 25% of post-aborted women had consulted psychiatrists as compared with 3% in the control group. Particularly at risk were teenagers, divorced women and those who had had multiple terminations.

Finally, it must be remembered that deaths from abortion still occur, particularly in such countries as Romania and Russia. The best statistical results come from Finland which found that women who abort are approximately four times more likely to die in the following year than those who carry their pregnancies to term. At the expense of repetition it is worth restating the fact that the principal causes of abortion related maternal death within a week of surgery are **haemorrhage**, **infection**, **embolism**, **anaesthesia**, and **undiagnosed ectopic pregnancy**. Indeed, in the United States abortion is reported to be the fifth leading cause of maternal death, although not usually reported as such.

I have just recorded what those who promote abortion call "safe, legal abortions"; but the majority of abortions are performed on healthy young women, and abortionists rarely explain the health risks to their patients.

No Safe Abortions

There is no such thing as "a safe legal abortion." Abortion is a decriminalized crime against humanity.

Epilogue

The purpose of writing this book was to take the reader on a journey of discovery. The stories are gathered from my thirty-seven years of gynaecological practice, although a few occurred at an earlier stage when I was in training.

Many of those stories deal with life-shattering and life-changing experiences that patients shared with me, and they include some, which patients begged me to write down and publish so that others might learn from their mistakes. Thus, they are particularly precious and are completely different from the normal medical articles and research papers that doctors write, for the latter contain dry information and statistics from which all emotional and speculative information has been strictly removed. I did at one stage attempt to keep statistics by giving all my patients a questionnaire to fill in, but soon abandoned it as it did not provide any in depth answers to the overriding question as to why women choose to have abortions.

I have, as far as I could, refrained from giving my own opinion about the patients' individual decisions but have, at the end of many of the stories, given current medical information relating to the medical conditions mentioned so that readers may be made aware of the latest medical research on the topics mentioned. During my medical career I have trained in several gynaecological sub-specialties: infertility, microsurgery, in vitro fertilization, and laser surgery, and have come across complications of the abortion scene in all of these disciplines.

During medical training you learn many things that remain for the rest of your life, but some also create dilemmas of which resuscitation is one.If you are a boy scout or a girl guide you are taught first-aid and resuscitation. In medical school you learn more, but as a junior doctor the training in resuscitation is all important for you never know when you will be faced with the necessity to commence treating a patient with cardiac arrest (cessation of the heart beat) before others, more experienced than yourself, arrive on the scene, since the first three minutes are vital if treatment is to succeed.

In our London hospital the number called when a patient was suspected of having developed cardiac arrest was 2222. On hearing that number anything that you were doing was abandoned and you ran, breathless and with adrenaline (a hormone secreted by the adrenal gland causing muscular action, stimulation and excitement) pumping, to the scene to attempt to save life. You commenced cardio-pulmonary resuscitation (resuscitation of heart and lungs) immediately. Only secondly, and usually when others had arrived, were signs of life looked for.

Yes, cardio-pulmonary resuscitation is fundamental teaching and training for all medical doctors these days. The guidelines are reviewed and regularly revised by the Royal College of Anaesthetists, the Royal College of Physicians and the Resuscitation Council (UK), and they publish a joint statement on cardio-pulmonary resuscitation: "Standards for Clinical Practice and Training". Depending on circumstances and what is available to hand, the one overriding principle is to start resuscitation immediately, while those who arrive later check for signs of life or death.

What are the signs of death? As with all medical advances these signs have changed or developed over the years. In Classical Greek and Roman society signs of death were: absence of heart beat, absence of respiration and onset of putrefaction. In

Mediaeval times a lighted candle was held to the mouth and a flicker of the candle flame confirmed that the person was still alive. In 1742 John Bruhier recorded fifty-two examples of supposed live burials in his book, "L'incertitude des signes de la mort." Since then more rigorous methods have been employed to make sure that an apparently dead person is truly dead.

In hospital these days if a nurse finds an unresponsive patient with absent respiration, absent pulse and fixed, dilated pupils she commences resuscitation and sends for medical help. Resuscitation is continued while an electro-cardiogram (record of electrical waves generated by the heart beat) and an electro-encephalogram (record of electrical impulses inside the brain) are recorded. However, resuscitation should still be continued and investigation for the vital signs repeated.

I remember as a young doctor being called in the middle of the night to an old man with advanced cancer who was not expected to live for many more months and who had developed cardiac arrest. Resuscitation was successful and the old gentleman was truly grateful, in spite of the fact that he was suffering much pain on account of his disease. For life is sweet, or as Shakespeare says through the mouth of Hamlet:

> But that the dread of something after death,
> The undiscovered country from whose bourn
> No traveller returns, puzzles the will,
> And makes us rather bear those ills we have
> Than fly to others we know not of?

On the following morning, although exhausted by the drama of the previous night, I was busy seeing patients in the Gynaecological Out Patients' Clinic. There I saw a woman who was complaining of amenorrhoea (absent periods). She proved to be 18 weeks pregnant and an ultrasound confirmed this. I showed her the baby's movements and heart beat and also indicated that he was suffering from a bout of hiccups. The patient was unimpressed. She said that the pregnancy had not been planned and she requested termination. I was shocked! All the signs of life were present here. Here too was a baby with a full life ahead of him, while I had spent half the previous night resuscitating an old man with hardly any signs of life, and who had, at best, only a few weeks or months to live. Then I remembered something in the guidelines issued by the Royal College of Obstetricians and Gynaecologists. It advised the use of common sense. Yes, I would use common sense. I was not a computer. There was no life-threatening condition that indicated that I should recommend termination. Request refused!

Another of the dilemmas that had puzzled me during my years of fretting over the problem of termination of pregnancy was that of responsibility. I discussed this on one occasion with a patient of mine who claimed that she was pro-choice and pro-abortion. I mentioned that one needed to have respect for human life and for the living; but she replied that nothing that could not exist independently could be considered to be human life. She then, as an after-thought, went on to say, "I don't want to be responsible for somebody else." I thought, what muddled, if not hypocritical, reasoning she has. First of all she implies that a foetus is not human because it is dependent for it's life on its mother, and then she admits that the real reason that she wishes to have an abortion is because she is unwilling to be responsible for her baby."

Down the ages we have fought for freedom, and even children, once they approach maturity, wish to escape from parental control. In reality, however, we are all dependent on each other, and this is particularly so in civilized countries. A woman seeks contraception, but the pill or the Intra-Uterine Contraceptive Device (IUCD) is made by some pharmaceutical company that sells it to a hospital or chemist from whom it is purchased by the patient. If she has sexual relations with a man and becomes pregnant she is dependent on a midwife or obstetrician to look after her during the pregnancy and to deliver her, and even if she has an abortion she is still dependent on the gynaecologist to carry it out. We only need to look at a developing country to see how enormous is the maternal and foetal mortality. Every second some woman in the world dies in childbirth or as the result of abortion. In other words, we are all dependent on each other and, in many instances, our very lives depend on someone else. Not many would survive on a desert island! Even in the United Kingdom maternal mortality was still high in 1928, but now, with the advances in maternal care it is low, although deaths still do occur from time to time.

I remember that some forty years ago when I was writing my MD thesis on Poliomyelitis, the hospitals were all full of paralysed patients dependent on the nursing staff for care, and on Iron Lungs to enable them to breath. My attention on one occasion was taken by a young man of twenty-eight whose only part of his body that he could move was his big toe. With that he was learning to paint in the hope that he could become an artist.

Nowadays in hospitals we see people with kidney failure dependent on dialysis or on the donation of a kidney from someone else for their very life. Even the woman sitting in front of me was dependent on the medical profession. How could I convince her that dependency does not take away the joy or meaning of being human?

Our independence should be increased by improving that which makes us dependent. Just consider the premature baby. A baby who weighs between 1,500 and 2,500 gm is said to be premature. Not so long ago any born weighing less than 1,000 gm was sure to die. We now have life support systems sufficient to care for babies weighing 400 gm. Research workers are now studying the dynamics of the placenta with the hope of being able to make an artificial one capable of sustaining babies of much smaller weight. We only have to look at In Vitro Fertilization to see what has already been achieved. An egg can now be fertilized and allowed to divide outside the human body.

The foetus is not a passive, dependent, nerveless, fragile vegetable as tradition has implied but a young human being: dynamic, plastic, resilient, who is, in very large measure, in charge of his environment and destiny. For the duration of pregnancy it is the foetus, not the mother, who initiates all the changes that make his mother a suitable host for himself. This newly conceived embryo supplies all the hormones necessary for maintenance of the decidua (the lining of the uterus in pregnancy). In fact he changes all his mother's physiology in order to ensure his survival. In other words it is the mother, not the foetus, who is passive and dependent. One cannot understand the physiology of pregnancy if one remains in ignorance of the dominant partner in the relationship, namely the foetus.

Medical techniques are always subject to change. Old obstetric books were written with the care of the mother in mind. Little thought was given to the needs of the foetus; while for the baby who was too large to pass through the maternal birth canal a destructive operation on the baby was always possible. Then came the advances in medical technology following the Second World War: better anaesthetic techniques, blood transfusion, improvement in surgical techniques, all of which eliminated the fear of Caesarean section.

Nowadays every woman expects to give birth to a perfect baby, consequently the work of the Obstetrician and Paediatrician now start at fertilization. The time when the Paediatrician's first contact with the baby occurred when he was handed the baby after the delivery is long past. The list of foetal diseases that can be diagnosed and treated in one-way or another steadily grows. Foetal medicine is now a separate specialty. Not all of us will live to be old, but each of us was once a foetus!

The majority of pregnancies are uncomplicated and result in the birth of normal, healthy babies. However, some require additional care for the unborn baby or foetus, and demand the attention of paediatricians especially skilled in such care, nowadays called foetologists or perinatologists.

Diagnostic skills concerned with foetal disease have improved enormously in recent years, so much so that medical congresses and symposia are now regularly held to consider the 'foetus as a patient'. Therapeutic approaches, of course, are still limited. Perhaps the most significant advance is that professionals and patients, too, now consider the foetus to be a separate individual and a potential patient in his own right.

Various organizations and societies for the study of perinatology have been formed to engage in research. They have already contributed enormously to our understanding of foetal medicine. This has led to the investigation of babies in utero, and promises to enable such specialists to treat some foetal abnormalities while the baby is still within its mother's womb rather than suggesting that they should be aborted. Indeed, some such operations have already been successfully performed. This type of sub-specialty has sparked the imagination of paediatricians around the world so that now the teaching of foetal medicine has even been taken up with enthusiasm by some doctors in developing countries

One often hears the 'politically correct' cavilling at Roman Catholic and other religious leaders for trying to foist their morality on others. Indeed, I even came across it in a writers' group when I dared to utter the word, 'morality'. However, abortion is not merely a religious, sectarian or even a private morality problem. It is no less than a question of the civil right to life. If you or I have the civil right to life then is it not the duty of all citizens in the pluralistic society in which we now live, regardless of the religion, faith, or private moral sensitivity of its members to protect the unborn child's civil rights? If you recognize the woman's right to the possession and control of her own person, then surely you must recognize the same for her unborn child to the possession and control of his or her own person?

I am in a dilemma and keep asking myself why a so-called civilized society has become so threatened by its own offspring that it seeks the violence of human abortion to relieve its anxiety. Why do innocent children become such a threat to their parents that they are moved to destroy them? Why does not society, which attempts to promote peace and justice, realise that it is actually promoting the opposite?

My own experience of dealing with this problem of requests for abortion over many years enabled me, with the help of counsellors, psychiatrists, lawyers, yes, and even clergy, to encourage about 50% of those women whom I saw happily to carry on with their pregnancies. Some of those patients whom I had the pleasure to see some ten, or even fifteen, years later, remarkable as it may seem, said that those unwanted children had become their most prized possessions! Of the others, some 25% came bitterly to regret what they had done. This is in keeping with a report that I read recently that said that 31% of patients interviewed who underwent termination of abortion lived to regret their actions. Sadly the medical, counselling and legal professions have been very negligent in providing help to such people in their hour of need. Many, if not most, immediately acquiesce to the the woman's cry for abortion without attempting to take an in depth history to decide whether or not it is in the woman's best interest, let alone, dare I say, to even mention the child that she is carrying.

As noted at the beginning of this book I wanted as a young woman to fight for women's rights because, even then, although men paid lip-service for the requirement of men to care first for women and children, especially during war, nevertheless they still looked upon women as the weaker sex whose job was essentially that of looking after the home and family, in spite of the fact that most of them were also in fulltime employment. I too wanted to help to improve the lot of women. I was not a member of the Women's Liberation Movement, nor did I wish to exacerbate the battle of the sexes, but as a young student I really thought that pregnancy, childbirth and abortion were problems that should be dealt with and settled by women.

After finishing at medical school I chose to specialize in Obstetrics and Gynaecology because I believed that since I was a woman I could better understand the needs of women than could my male colleagues. I asked myself how could any man understand what it was like to start a pregnancy, or care for a baby. How could he appreciate the fear, anguish, or worry that a woman felt when first conscious that she was pregnant? No man suffers from vomiting in pregnancy, nor has he to continue working in his chosen profession while trying, at the same time, to care for a baby. I appreciate that at that stage of my life I was as ignorant about such things as were my fellow male doctors, nevertheless, I convinced myself that I knew better, and for the reasons that I have mentioned, I thought I could understand why women were trying to get termination of pregnancy legalized.

At the beginning my knowledge of embryology and intrauterine life were rudimentary, but gradually, as I learnt more, I came to realise that I was caring equally for two people. This slow realisation of the worth of all people is confirmed by history, that is, until the 1967 Abortion Act was passed. Thus, the strong built their reputation and amassed their fortunes by oppressing the weak. The black man served his master who considered him of no account, except in so far as he was able to gather in his sugar cane crop, or whatever else he instructed him to do. We are this year celebration the two hundredth anniversary of the year in which the slave trade was banned; although, as everyone knows, there are still millions of virtual slaves around the world, many more, in fact, than there were when slavery was banned. This indeed mirrors the abortion scandal, for many more babies are now being legally aborted around the world than were ever destroyed by back street abortionists.

What, indeed, are the rights of children? Besides the normal rights of all human beings children were granted the rights to special protection because of their vulnerability to exploitation and abuse, and in 1989 the United Nations General Assembly adopted the convention on the Rights of the Child which has been ratified by 191 countries throughout the world at the last count. Previously in 1959 the General Assembly of the United Nations passed a Declaration of the Rights of the Child that said, "The child, by reason of his physical and mental immaturity needs special safeguards and care, including appropriate legal protection, before as well as after birth." Sadly, the latest legal rights of the child passed by the United Nations in 1989 expunged the legal rights previously granted in 1959 to the unborn child.

I here include some of the questions of patients, who either requested or who had had abortions throughout the years, and my replies. Much is repetitive but it is needful if we are adequately to investigate this problem. Perhaps first, however, I should mention the reply that the patient, whose letter I included towards the end of the book, gave when I, contrary to my usual practice, acted the part of an advocate of abortion. "Why shouldn't a woman have the right to chose an abortion?" I queried. "In the same way that it is not right for her to abuse her own child or carry out infanticide," she immediately replied. To her, who had in the past had a termination, it was now quite obvious that the foetus within was a separate being, her own child no less.

Another patient of mine posed the question that all those who are pro-choice say they believe, but which she, at least, had the humility to ask. "How can a foetus be a human being when it has no separate existence? Surely it must be part of the woman's body?" My answer was that advances in medical science have proved beyond reasonable doubt that the human embryo or foetus is biologically separate from its mother from the moment of conception. This individual must be human. Human beings can only conceive human beings, just as elephants can only conceive elephants. The placenta, amniotic fluid, cord and support system are all made by the baby and are biologically separate from its mother. In Vitro Fertilization shows that the embryo can develop outside the female body; and medical science is steadily inventing a means of survival so that very small premature babies can still develop outside and apart from the mother. Furthermore, should a patient come to me and ask me to remove part of her body the law forbids me to do so. If then the foetus is part of the human body I am forbidden to obey her and perform an abortion! After all, we all hear of desperate people who need money and try to sell one of their kidneys; but we know that the law forbids the sale of organs for money, so they are unsuccessful in their quest. No educated person doubts that the embryo or foetus is alive and is human, although some may argue as to whether or not he is a person. If he is a person then under law he has the same rights as you or I, the elderly, the disabled, or infants. In the United States in the late 1800s black people had their personhood revoked so that slave owners were allowed by law, if need be, to kill their slaves; while in the early 1900s in Canada women were still not considered to be persons and it took the historic Person's Case to have women awarded the right to be considered 'persons' under the law. In Nazi Germany of course only sixty years or so ago Jews were declared to be non-persons and so had no rights.

My husband, when a junior doctor, worked in a famous London Teaching Hospital whose world renowned Radiologist had perfected the art of taking four X rays of a woman's pelvis by which means he was able to forecast those that would have difficulty in childbirth. So expert had he become that in the patients who had pelvic abnormalities he could forecast what kind of complications would arise during labour and what type of intrauterine manipulation and forceps delivery would be needed to overcome the abnormality. This gave the hospital a great reputation around the world.

However, a research worker in the Department of Preventive Medicine in Oxford, Alice Stewart by name, had in 1955 been alerted to the numbers of children dying of leukaemia, so she persuaded local health officials around the country to interview the mothers of more than one and a half thousand children who had died from leukaemia during the previous two years. A similar number of mothers and children were used as controls, and it soon became apparent that twice as many cancer deaths had occurred amongst children below the age of ten whose mothers had received a series of X-rays while pregnant.

This finding was not well received by departments of radiology throughout the country for it was believed that radiation exposure at the level given was quite safe. The dispute smouldered on for more than five years until her work was finally confirmed by a much larger series from the Harvard School of Public Health. With this confirmatory evidence from America the Radiology Departments around the country that specialised in X-rays used for diagnostic purposes in maternity hospitals fell apart, for although such consultants in those departments were helping to prevent women from having long and unfruitful labours, yet their very methods were having disastrous results on the unborn child. Cannot this be compared with the disastrous results that termination is having on our unborn generations? More than this however: Had Radiologists persisted in taking antenatal X-rays of the mother and foetus they could have been taken to court by either the mother or the baby after he had been born, if harm had occurred. I am now retired but I am required by law to keep all my obstetric notes for twenty-one years so that they are available should any problem arise in the developing child and he or she thinks that it has been caused by my negligence while he or she was in utero (within the uterus).

Even the argument put forward by the pro-choice lobby that liberalization of abortion ensures that every child born is a wanted child is shown to be false; for during the last three years, when numbers of abortions have never been higher, the images of serious child abuse online has quadrupled, according to figures from Britain's internet watchdog recently published. Indeed, another study reports that 90% of battered children were from wanted pregnancies. A lack of caring is a flaw in the person who ought to care, not in the person who ought to be cared for. Thus, we return to the question of whether or not the unborn is a fully human person, not whether he or she is, or is not, wanted; and I think we have already proved conclusively that the unborn child is a full human being right from the time of conception.

Abortion, it was said, would solve the problem of the unwanted child, as well as many of the other social and psychological evils of society. In fact it has done nothing in this respect. It has merely created further physical, psychological and ethical problems that have left a permanent scar on modern society.

Some may argue that the writing is emotive. Of course it is! How could it be otherwise in a subject where the patient's emotions are, in almost every case, a prime factor which brings the patient to the doctor to request abortion. The woman sitting in front of me is a woman full of fears and doubts, battling against the mentally clouding effects of rising hormone levels, often with accompanying vomiting. She needs understanding. She needs sympathy. Often she wants someone else to make decisions for her. A request for abortion is a cry for help!

I have learnt much over the years from my patients. They have been amongst my greatest teachers. It is my desire that, likewise, they may be able to enlighten the reader. High school children may rebel against learning something that is dead and past, and, although the schoolteacher may hold to an opposite view, nevertheless, a beneficent government acquiesces to their demands. It is indeed fortunate that television has allowed historians to portray their periods of historical expertise and so keep alive national and world history for the common man. The wise statesman or politician, of course, does study history and uses the knowledge thus gained to discern a moral responsibility to protect his nation and fellow men from harm. Plato, I believe, it was, who argued that those who tell stories rule society, and perhaps the most important stories are those told by the ones who have actually had a life changing experience and are brave enough to share it with others.

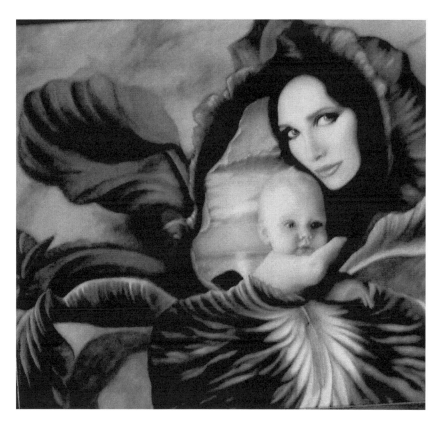

Painted by Audrey Sanders in 1992.

Mother, You filled my days with rain-bow lights,
Fairytales and sweet dream nights,
A kiss to wipe away my tears,
Gingerbread to ease my fears.
You gave the gift of life to me,
And then in love, you set me free.
I thank you for your tender care,
For deep warm hugs and being there.
I hope that when you think of me,
A part of you, you'll always see.
                    Anonymous